HOW TO BE YOUR DOCTOR'S FAVORITE PATIENT

And Get the Care You Deserve

Brad Colegate, MD

Published by FastPencil, Inc.

Copyright © 2010 Brad Colegate

Published by FastPencil, Inc.
3131 Bascom Ave.
Suite 150
Campbell CA 95008 USA
(408) 540-7571
(408) 540-7572 (Fax)
info@fastpencil.com
http://www.fastpencil.com

Illustrated by Jim Caputo

No part of this publication may be reproduced, stored in a retrieval system, or transmitted, in any form, or by any means, electronic, mechanical, photocopying, recording, or otherwise, without the prior consent of the publisher.

The Publisher makes no representations or warranties with respect to the accuracy or completeness of the contents of this book and specifically disclaim any implied warranties of merchantability or fitness for a particular purpose. Neither the publisher nor author shall be liable for any loss of profit or any commercial damages.

*This book is dedicated to all patients.
Thank you for your patience!*

Contents

Acknowledgements ix
    Note to the Reader ix
Introduction xi
1. PERSONALITIES 1
    Trekkies 1
    The Social Caller 4
    The Silent Type 6
    The Pierced Patient 8
    The Macho Man 10
    The Executive 13
    The Violent Patient 15
    The Name-Caller 17
    The White Glove Patient 19
    Patients Who Don't Like Doctors 21
    The Self-Destructing Patient 23
    "Special" Patients 25
    The Lawyer 27
    The Queen of Extraneous Details 29
    The Medical Student 31
    The Physician 33
2. TIME & MONEY 35
    "I Have This Form For You To Fill Out" 36
    Staff Members 39
    "I Don't Have Time To Be Sick" 41
    "Just Phone It In" 43
    The Impatient Patient 46
    The Laundry List 48
    The Deadbeat 50

The Referral Refuser 52

"Call Me" 54

"Oh, By The Way, Doc…" 56

The Powder Room Patient 58

3. FAMILY TROUBLES 59

    The Menace 60

    The Family Member 62

    Dr. Mom 64

    The Silent Partner 66

    The Family Entourage 68

    The Teenager's Warden 70

4. THE SEEKERS 73

    The Siren 74

    The Vitamin Junkie 76

    The Drug Seeker 78

    The Doctor Shopper 80

    The New Guru 82

    Ponce De Leon 85

    The Doctor Idolizer 87

    "Please Excuse Johnny From School Today" 89

    The Antibiotic Addict 91

5. MISCELLANEOUS MISUNDERSTANDINGS 94

    The Waiting Room Magazine Bandit 95

    "I'm Allergic To Something" 98

    "It's A Little White Pill…" 100

    The Handshaker 101

    The Soap Opera 103

    The Fashion Model 105

    "My Chiropractor Says…" 107

The Sensitive Stomach	109
Ring-A-Ding-Ding	111
"You Want To Do What?!"	113
The Animal Lover	115
Patients Who Die	117
Playtime In The Office	119
Patients Who Don't Follow Up	121
"Have I Got News For You!"	123
The Refrigerated Stethoscope	125
"Have You Ever Had This Problem, Doctor…"	127
"Oh, My Aching Back"	129
The Patient Who Plays Doctor	131
6. Postscript	133
7. About the Author	134
8. About the Illustrator	135

Acknowledgements

This book has been in my head for many years, but bringing it to fruition has involved a number of other level-headed and talented people. Thanks to my nephew, James Lake; my partner, Andrew Mitchell; and Emily Seligman for their sharp-eyed reviews and editorial advice. Thanks to all the people at FastPencil for their assistance with the publishing of this book, and to Jim Caputo for his wonderful illustrations.

Note to the Reader
The characters in this book are entirely fictional (with the exception of the author himself in one story), and any resemblance to persons living or dead is purely coincidental. The stories and the advice which follows them are general in nature and may not apply to your particular situation. As always, consult with your own physicians regarding any specific questions or concerns about your health and medical care.

Introduction

"If you've got your health, you've got everything," it's been said, and we, as a nation, are eagerly seeking to fulfill that dictum. We join health clubs, take yoga classes, and buy vitamin supplements, at a yearly cost of billions of dollars, but we often overlook one of the most important links to good health: our relationships with our physicians. But improving these relationships can help us achieve better health–and there's no additional office charge!

On average, we visit a physician nearly three times per year, for a whopping total of 800 million office visits per year. That might make you think that Americans love seeing their doctors–but it's often a love-hate relationship. More and more people are voicing their dissatisfaction with the traditional medical system and turning to alternative therapies such as acupuncture, homeopathy, and chiropractic. Still, most medical care takes place in a traditional office setting, and patients themselves have the power to increase their level of satisfaction with their care providers–and their level of health–by following some simple suggestions on what to do (and not to do) in the doctor's office.

We have bought millions of books to help us get along better with our spouses, children, and in-laws, and yet very little has been written about the doctor-patient relationship–the foundation for receiving good care–or the ingredients that are needed to make this relationship work. Relationships are largely abstract and emotional, but the behaviors they involve can be defined and illustrated. Bear in mind that the doctor-patient relationship involves two human beings–(yes, doctors are human, too)–and that getting what you want out of any relationship involves responsibilities and seeing the other person's point of view.

We've learned that if we don't treat our spouses well, we're not even going to get to first base when it comes to getting the love we want; respect, openness, and affection will make us winners at home. Likewise, if we have difficulties in the way we deal with our doctors, those difficulties will become roadblocks to getting the care we deserve. The premise of this book is that you will be better served, happier, and healthier if you get along well with your doctor, perhaps more so than if you receive any particular test, drug, or treatment.

Using colorful vignettes drawn from my years of experience in primary care (but using fictional patients and physicians), this book illustrates many of the challenges that test the doctor-patient relationship. Each scene will be followed by an analysis and advice as to what could be done to improve the situation. By following these guidelines, you can become "your doctor's favorite patient"–and get the care you deserve!

PERSONALITIES

Trekkies

Jayvon Jackson hardly looked up when the doctor walked into the room; he was too busy playing the computer game he got for Christmas to notice. Having just passed Level 4, he was waging "The Ultimate Battle" on Level 5. He had learned all the tricks to the weapons in his arsenal, and they had made him the all-powerful master of this cyber-planet.

But on Planet Earth, he wasn't invulnerable. The previous week he had come to the doctor's office after feeling dizzy for three days. Dr. Jenna Brooks examined him but wasn't sure what was causing his symptoms. When the physician ordered a panel of blood tests, Jayvon was certain it would reveal the answer to his diagnostic dilemma. So, on his follow-up visit, he was more than a little surprised when the Dr. Brooks now told him, "Your tests are all normal—no clues there."

"What? You still don't know what's wrong?" he asked incredulously. "How about doing a CT scan, or an MRI?"

"If your symptoms persist, we may need to consider that, but I doubt it would be helpful, considering your normal neurological exam."

"You mean to tell me, with all the tests you guys can do nowadays, you can't always figure out what's goin' on?"

"Yes," said Dr. Brooks with a sigh, "I'm afraid so."

"Oh, man. Guess I was born a century too early."

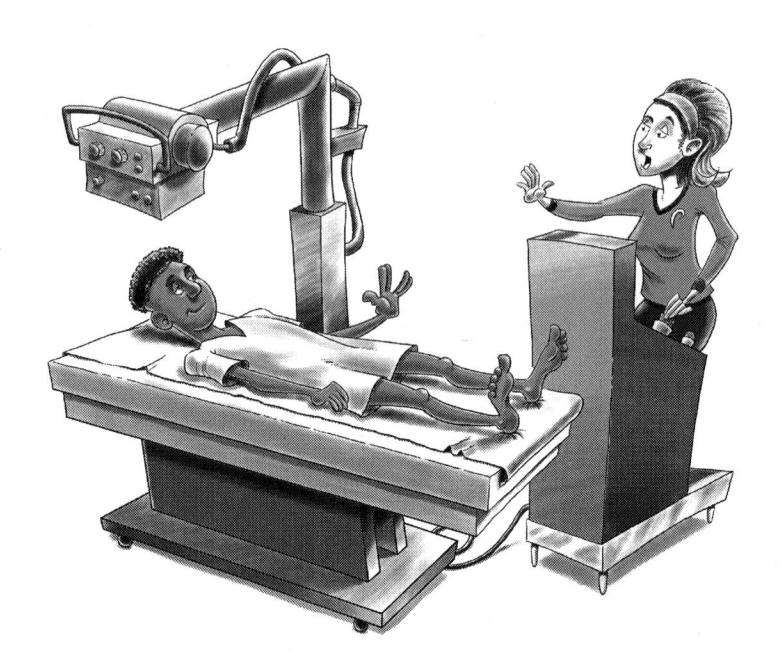

"Hold still, and we'll have the diagnosis in 2.7 seconds!"

Science fiction is fascinating–a tantalizing look at what our future might someday hold–but it is still a fiction. We've all been enthralled by the *Star Wars* and *Star Trek* movies and television programs, and in a universe of intergalactic travel, it seems that anything is possible. But you don't have to look too closely to see that those characters who conquer worlds can't seem to conquer their own wrinkles or baldness.

To someone born a hundred years ago, the medical world of today might seem as fantastic as those movies. Medical technology, like computer, aviation, and other technologies, is doing things that once were only a dream. Sometimes all the new hardware gives us a false sense of security and shields us from the hard fact that people get sick and die–eventually. This isn't to say that we shouldn't use technology to our advantage, but that like any other resource, we need to recognize its limits, conserve it, and use it when appropriate.

- *Do* expect your physician to order blood tests or imaging studies in evaluating unusual symptoms; sometimes they can help to pinpoint the diagnosis.

- *Don't* expect technology to provide the diagnosis and treatment. Medicine is still as much of an art as it is a science, and there still are humans behind the machines.

- *Don't* demand extensive testing as part of a routine check-up. Only a very few tests (such as cholesterol) have proven to be worthwhile for screening purposes.

- *Do* ask for a second opinion if the testing goes on and on. A different human may find out more than the MRI machine.

- *Don't* smoke or engage in other unhealthy behaviors on the assumption that there will be a cure for lung cancer and other diseases twenty years from now—you may not live to see it!

The Social Caller

"Dr. Diogenes! Hello, my dear, how are you? I haven't seen you for ages!" exclaimed Mrs. Maureen O'Leary, the 63-year-old president of the Knoxtown Women's Auxiliary. "What have you been up to?" Anyone would think that the reason for her visit had nothing to do with any concern over her health, but rather a fascination with the whereabouts of her physician.

"Well, mostly I've been here at the office and the hospital," he replied. "And the little bit of time I have left I try to spend with my family."

"Oh, but I hope you and Jo won't be too busy to come to the Community Cabaret. It's going to be wonderful. I'm going to open the show—everyone simply insisted—with my version of 'Everything's Coming Up Roses.' People say I sound just like Ethel Merman. But of course you'll be there! I almost forgot your son Cody is appearing in *West Side Story*. Don't you wish our juvenile delinquents nowadays were still that tame?"

"Ah, yes. Now, tell me Mrs. O'Leary, what is it that brings you in today?"

"Oh, I suppose we do need to get back down to business. I just need a refill on my new blood pressure medicine. It's rather expensive, you know, though that's not a problem for me, but I can't see how most of your patients can afford to take it every day. It's no wonder some people are crying out for national health insurance, although that would be the ruination of our health care system as we know it, don't you think?"

"I'd love to have an opinion on that, but it seems the politicians are going to do what they want no matter what we doctors think. Your blood pressure was fine when the nurse took it, but let me just recheck it, and listen to your heart and lungs."

The silver-haired matron began chattering away again as Dr. Diogenes pumped up the blood pressure bulb. He put his finger to his lips, begging for silence, but it only shushed her for a moment. By the time she left with her new prescription in hand, the doctor realized he'd learned everything about her except her state of health. Indeed, it wasn't until her next visit, a month later, when she revealed, "We were so busy talking last time, doctor, that I forgot to tell you I've been having this nagging cough ever since I've been on this medication."

"I wish you'd have told me sooner," he admonished, but feeling a little guilty he hadn't uncovered this fact at the previous visit. The medication, a so-called ACE inhibitor, was doing an excellent job of lowering her blood pressure, but causing her cough. Fortunately, in this case the side effect was merely an annoyance, and the delay in reporting it to her physician resulted in no serious harm. Lucky for both of them!

Small talk can make a big difference in business settings. It can establish a sense of rapport and put people at ease, or provide a transition into weightier matters. Certainly in the setting of a physician's office, small talk can serve those functions, but in what is often a very limited amount of time, it can also distract from the matter at hand. While your physician should be friendly and be your ally, that's different from being social friends. In some small towns, a doctor may be social friends with many of his patients, but he still needs to keep his office a place of business.

- *Do* expect that your doctor will be friendly and may inquire into matters other than your health.

- *Don't* expect a large part of your visit to be taken up with social matters even if you're a friend as well as a patient. Call each other later at home!

The Silent Type

Forty-three-year-old Hagob Nararan hadn't been in to see his physician for several years, not since she removed a badly ingrown toenail from his right foot. Understandably, Dr. Debra Peters' first question to her patient was "What brings you back after all this time?"

"Just a check-up," he muttered.

Now Dr. Peters knew that someone who doesn't come in for several years is not the type of person to seek regular check-ups without having a problem, so she persevered by asking, "Are you sure that you're not having any particular health problems you need checked.?"

"No," he said, and continued to answer in monosyllables as she ran down her usual checklist of questions.

Soon, she'd finished both the history and physical exam and concluded, "Everything seems to be normal. It would be a good idea to do a cholesterol test on you though, as a screening measure."

"Okay."

"I'll write the order and then you can return anytime you'd like after you've been fasting for twelve hours, and we'll draw the blood. You can call two days after that for the result."

"Okay."

As she turned to leave him, he asked, "Will the blood test check for everything?"

"Well, no, it's just a cholesterol level. There are hundreds of different blood tests."

"Oh."

"Is there something you're worried about that you'd like checked?"

"No. Well, yes. What about HIV?"

After much beating around the bush, Dr. Peters was able to ascertain that Mr. Nararan was worried about an encounter he had with a female prostitute while away on a business trip a few months ago. Although a widower, he was still tormented by the thought that he had dishonored his late wife by having sex with a hooker–and felt sure he'd be punished by catching HIV.

When the results came back negative in a few days, Mr. Nararan smiled and became effusive in his relief. "Thank you, thank you. Dr. Peters, you have made me so happy. I will be sure to see you whenever I have a problem."

"Next time," advised Dr. Peters, "just tell me what's on your mind."

Doctors aren't mind readers; they base their diagnoses on the things their patients *tell* them. The less information they have, the more difficult it is to arrive at a correct diagnosis. Doctors will generally keep probing until they feel they have enough information. Of course, too much extraneous information can be bad, too. For example, in response to the question "When did you start having abdominal pain?" one could hear the following responses:

"A while ago." (Too little info.)

"It started two weeks ago while I was just sitting on the couch reading." (About right.)

"It started at 8:15 p.m. last Thursday while I was reading this new murder mystery, *Black Ice*, by Duane Patterson. He's my favorite author." (Too much!)

Some information, such as sexual concerns, may be difficult for you to talk about, but remember: your physician is your confidante. Besides, you won't shock her–there's probably nothing you can tell her that she hasn't heard before (or at least read about in medical school).

- *Do* tell the doctor the real reason you're there.
- *Don't* just answer "yes" or "no" to all your doctor's questions.
- *Do* volunteer information that you think might be helpful.
- *Don't* keep secrets from your doctor when they relate to your problem.
- *Do* expect confidentiality to be respected.

The Pierced Patient

Gillian Landers couldn't wait to get away to college–or perhaps more accurately, away from the parents who controlled every aspect of her life. Two hundred miles and three hours away from her small town, she was free now–free to party, to play–and get pierced. She'd been wanting to get her belly-button pierced ever since she saw a model in *Elle* with a gold-and-emerald ring in her mid-section. Her mother had let her get her earlobes pierced, of course, but that was nothing special, and both her parents had thrown a fit when she said she wanted her belly-button done.

It didn't hurt much when the guy at "The Nifty Needle" did it–he was a pro who did his work as easily and as casually as a seamstress darning a sock. But two days later it began to be painful, and pus was oozing from the puncture site. By the time she sheepishly made her way to the doctor's office in another two days, there was also redness and swelling for an inch all the way around the ring.

"I'll put you on an antibiotic, but that ring's going to have to come out, at least until this is all healed," advised Dr. Lois Gavin. "Otherwise, it acts as a hiding place for the bacteria."

Gillian burst into tears. "I should have listened to my mother. She told me it would get infected." Composing herself, she continued, "I don't want this to happen again. Would you do the piercing for me next time, doctor?"

"No," she said, "I don't do piercing."

"Why not?"

"Because it's really a *cosmetic*, not a medical, procedure."

"I think maybe you don't want to because you're like my parents and you think it's weird."

"Well, I do happen to think the human body looks better without any extra holes in it."

Body-piercing is a practice that has become very popular, especially among teenagers and college students. For some, it's a wild new fashion, a bold declaration of nonconformity. Arguments against it range from the aesthetic: "it's ugly"; to the practical: "how does he blow his nose with that thing in?"; to the moralistic: "it's mutilating your God-given body." From a medical standpoint, there are no *advantages* to piercing (one doesn't absorb iron into the blood from a steel ring, for instance), but there are certain risks, and therefore many physicians are against the practice. The pain caused by the procedure is highly subjective; many claim after a piercing that "it didn't hurt at all."

Bleeding can be a problem if the site isn't chosen properly, and keloid formation (excessive scarring) can occur in some individuals. Infection is the main risk–not so much from the piercer (although certainly it's important for the piercer to use proper hygiene and technique)—but rather from your own skin bacteria invading the wounded flesh. So, if you have a piercing done, keep the site scrupulously clean until (and even after) it has healed. But if complications develop, don't be afraid to see your doctor; she'll help you get better—even if she does give you a "piercing look" of admonishment.

- *Do* carefully select a qualified piercer before you get any piercing done.
- *Don't* get pierced in a drunken or drug-induced state, or you may agree to something you'll regret when you're sober.
- *Do* see your doctor right away if signs of infection appear.
- *Do* expect *not* to get a lecture on the "evils" of piercing.

The Macho Man

"How's it goin', doc?" asked Dave Carter as he extended his beefy hand to Dr. Jess Heinz, who accepted it and got a no-nonsense, bone-crunching shake. This security guard was accustomed to using his handshake to transmit a sense of his strength and establish his territory–not to show mere friendliness. "You know, doc," he said, as if using the familiar and diminutive form of address to keep Dr. Heinz in his place, "I'm starting to lose a lot of hair, and I wonder if I could get some of those pills to make it grow back. It doesn't matter to me, of course, but women seem to like hair."

It was a simple problem and a simple request, and Dr. Heinz, a busy man most days and especially so today, did not try to delve further into the matter. Handing Mr. Carter a prescription, he said, "It doesn't work for everybody, but what the heck, you can give it a try."

As the physician was heading out the door, Mr. Carter asked, "Do you think we should do a testosterone check first, doc?"

"Why do you ask?"

"Well, I was just thinking, maybe, uh, I don't have enough in my system and that's why my hair's falling out."

"If low testosterone were the cause, women would all be bald."

"But, uh, wouldn't it be a good idea to check it anyway?"

Dr. Heinz looked his patient in the eye and said firmly, but with a smile, "Look, Dave, I want to help you, but I don't have time for all this beating around the bush. What's the real problem?"

"Sorry. It's just kinda hard to talk about. I've been having trouble lately getting an erection."

So after further discussion (which revealed that Mr. Carter was also urinating excessively and losing weight) and a blood sugar test, the man who almost left the office with a diagnosis of male-pattern baldness left with a diagnosis of diabetes with secondary erectile dysfunction.

How to be Your Doctor's Favorite Patient • 11

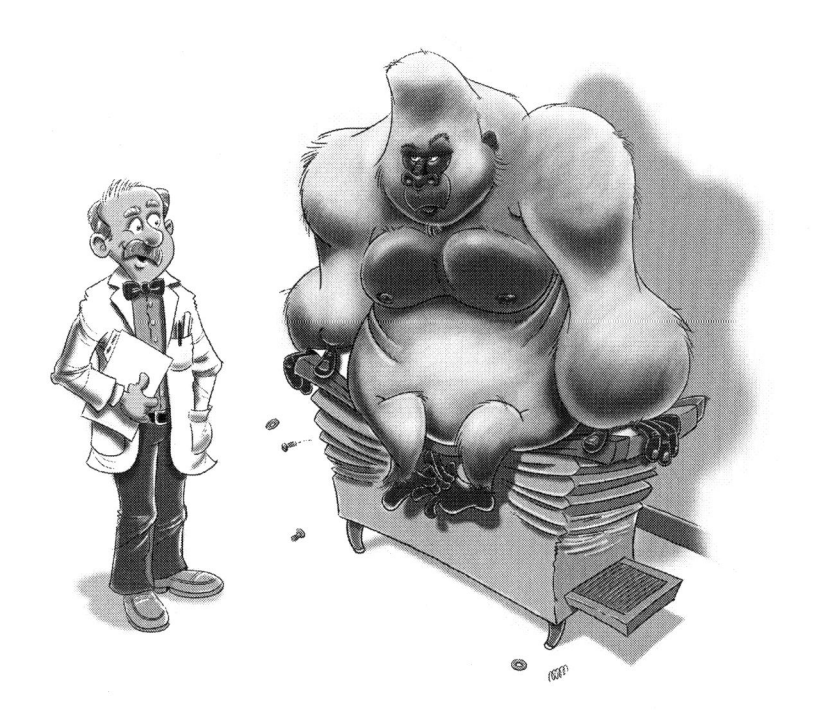

"I think we'd better check your testosterone level today."

Male-bashing has become a popular, even accepted, practice nowadays. Men's sexist domination existed for so long (still exists?) that knocking them down a few pegs doesn't seem unfair, and many of them try to "take it like a man." Even as society is nearing gender equality for employment and other legally-mandated areas, some men cling stubbornly to behaviors that seem not only out-of-date but which can be harmful. Being a workaholic, drinking too much, and denying feelings (both emotional and physical pain) can have disastrous consequences for a man–or anybody.

Letting their guard down can be difficult for men to do, even in the presence of their physicians, who to some may seem to represent intimidating "father figures." Even if they view their doctors as allies, men often conceal things from their "buddies" for fear of appearing weak. Their relationships with their physicians then often suffer the same way their relationships with their loved ones do: from a lack of communication.

- *Do* tell your physician your intimate problems. Even if he does a complete physical, he still can't read your mind.

- *Don't* worry that the physician will laugh at you, and *do* expect him to show concern for you.

- *Don't* expect your physician to conspire with you in down-playing or overlooking a medical problem because you're afraid of it.

- *Do* see a male physician if you prefer, or

- *Do* consider seeing a female physician if that would make you feel more comfortable talking about certain issues.

The Executive

"Thanks for not keeping me waiting, Dr. Hadley," said the silver-haired gentleman seated in Exam Room 2, Mr. Alex Farmington. Sizing up her patient, Dr. Bernadette Hadley spied a tall, handsome man who was impeccably dressed from his gray silk Armani suit with dark blue Gregoria tie down to his custom-made black leather loafers.

"I've got a flight to New York in two hours," he said. "I think both of us know the importance of keeping on schedule."

"You probably do a better job of that than I do, I'm afraid," said Dr. Hadley, "but since you're the first patient on my schedule today, I don't have any excuse not to be on time."

Their conversation was interrupted by a series of high-pitched beeps. Dr. Hadley looked at her right hip, but her cell phone was silent.

"It's mine–the office," said Mr. Farmington. "Would you excuse me for just a moment?" he asked as he was already dialing. "Terry!" he shouted into the receiver. "Hold my calls til I get to the airport. I'll have to call them back on the flight." Turning to Dr. Hadley, he said, "Sorry. Back to the business at hand. I'm feeling great, but I'm due for a check-up. Sort of like my old Rolls-Royce—in perfect condition, but still in need of a tune-up now and then."

"Are there any particular things you're concerned about that you'd like to have checked?"

"Do it all—whatever needs to be done. Don't worry about the expense, of course."

"Fine. I'll do a physical, and then some tests, but there's really not a lot that needs to be done for the typical patient of your age who's feeling well."

"Excuse me, doctor, but I'm not your 'typical' patient."

"*My 'typical' patients aren't rich snobs,*" she thought, but said, "Yes, of course. Everyone has unique needs."

He seemed disappointed when at the end of the physical all she recommended was to check his cholesterol. "You had an extensive blood profile, ECG, and colonoscopy last year, all of which were normal, so there's really no point in repeating those things already."

"The colonoscopy I can do without, but as long as you're drawing blood, I'd like to have everything checked. I want all the bases covered."

"But..." she began.

"Just do it."

She gave in. "Okay. It's your money, or at least your insurer's money," she said, as she walked away feeling like one of his employees.

America is a society in which all of us are equal but everybody wants special treatment. Likewise, American medicine ostensibly tries to treat everyone the same based on their medical condition and not their pocketbooks–but fails. Even in countries like Britain which have socialized medicine, the rich are still able to purchase additional, specialized care.

When I was in training, there was even a special floor of the hospital where the well-heeled sick could recuperate with the aid of not only the nursing staff, but their own gourmet chef as well. Even though they paid extra for their privileges, this still seemed a little unfair to the rest of the patients who had to choke down their daily ration of broth and gelatin.

Rich people can be good patients, and there certainly are some doctors who cater to them: you can charge them more and expect to be paid. But there are limits to what your physician can do, no matter how much money you throw at her. Disease and death can only be bribed, not bought off altogether.

- *Do* realize that a champagne-and-caviar lifestyle may be a sign of privilege, but not of good health.
- *Don't* expect that your treatment will necessarily be any different than anyone else's with the same condition, regardless of income.
- *Do* realize that money can't buy happiness, love, or good health.

The Violent Patient

Dr. Dean Reitermann knew Martin Folsom was angry even before the patient began speaking: his uncombed morning hair stood out in mean porcupine-like spikes, his jaw was clenched with muscles that were visibly kneading across the bones, and his icy blue eyes glowered from behind glasses that sat slightly askew on his nose. With an optimistic smile, Dr. Reitermann extended his hand in a cheery greeting: "How are you today, Mr. Folsom? Nice to see you."

"Humph," he snorted. "Why don't you stop this damn buzzing in my ear? Then it'll be nice to see you."

Dr. Reitermann began to wonder if he should ask Lynn, his office nurse, to come into the room. But being 6' 2" and 200 pounds and having a black belt in karate made him confident that he need not be afraid of his slender young patient. "Let me take a look at you, then," the doctor said, and began to peer with his otoscope into Martin's left ear.

"What are you doing?" shouted Martin as he grabbed the physician's arm and pushed it away. "You're trying to plant some kind of radio in my head, aren't you?"

Dr. Reitermann glanced down at Martin's chart and now was reminded that the young man suffered from paranoid schizophrenia and was under the care of a psychiatrist. "Martin, have you been taking the medication that Dr. Carver prescribes for you?"

"Medication, medication, medication, medication," he chanted. "You and him are trying to poison me."

"No, of course not, we…"

But before the physician could finish his response, Martin snatched the chart from his hand and began ripping it up. "I'm destroying your plan!" he shouted.

Martin threw the shredded document into the doctor's face. "Stay away from me!" Martin yelled as he reached out his arm and with one sweep knocked the canisters off the equipment tray.

Shards of glass, wooden tongue blades, and cotton balls now littered the floor, and the noise of the crash brought Lynn into the room. "What's going on in here?" she asked as Martin ran past her.

"Nothing a little haloperidol won't fix," replied the shaken physician. A call to the patient's psychiatrist soon resulted in Martin's commitment to a hospital, until he was back on his medication and no longer a threat to others.

Violence in the workplace, while itself not common, is becoming a common source of anxiety among workers. Widely publicized incidents like an ex-postal employee who kills his former boss with an automatic weapon have made us all fearful for our own safety. A worker angry about being laid off, a customer spewing epithets over a defective product, or a colleague upset over a perceived insult can all trigger this fear.

Physicians and their staffs sometimes encounter verbal abuse from distraught patients, which can occasionally escalate into physical violence. In particular, physicians and clinic employees who perform abortions are terrified of this possibility. Regardless of one's stand on abortion, one has to condemn such violence. And just remember, if you should happen to have an altercation with your physician, he knows where your vital organs are located and how to get to them!

- *Do* remember that violence is not justified no matter how upset you are.
- *Do* discuss your feelings with your physician if you're upset about something.
- *Don't* be surprised if your doctor dismisses you as a patient if you've been verbally or physically abusive in the office.
- *Do* talk with a counselor or pastor if you continue to be angry with your doctor and his staff, rather than resort to violence. And, as a last resort, talk with your lawyer; while doctors hate to be sued, we'd rather be sued than shot.

The Name-Caller

Sheila Burnett was in a good mood. After a hectic summer, her kids were back in school, and she'd scheduled an all-afternoon spa treatment to pamper herself. All she had to do this morning was to get her annual Pap smear out of the way and then she'd be able to relax the rest of the day. A Ph. D. in chemistry who'd given up her career to focus on raising her three children, she decided she needed to focus on herself for a change. She'd found out that being a mother and a homemaker was sometimes delightful, sometimes maddening, and always challenging. Certainly she had as much respect now for all those other stay-at-home moms as she did for those charging ahead in the workplace. Her own degree didn't impress her as much as it used to, though it came in handy now and then when trying to figure out the reason for a culinary disaster or what cleaner to use on the bathtub scum.

The new physician she was meeting today was a woman about her own age (42), and she reminded Sheila of what path her life might have taken if she had stuck to pre-med in college instead of chemistry. "Good morning, Mrs. Burnett," said the physician. "I'm Dr. Kathy Isaacs. Nice to meet you."

"Hi, Kathy. It's nice to meet you, too. You don't mind if I call you 'Kathy,' do you?"

"No, not if you're more comfortable with that. You can call me Kathy, or you can call me Dr. Isaacs, just don't call me at two in the morning."

Sheila laughed and said, "Okay, and please drop the 'Mrs. Burnett'–it makes me sound too much like my mother-in-law. Considering my Ph.D., I suppose I could be 'Dr.' Burnett, but that's a bit pretentious."

"It's a deal," said Kathy, and the two women shook on it.

Names are a very important part of our identity. Even when burdened with a name like Eugene Periwinkle Borer, or tagged with the moniker of a long-deceased relative, we usually make peace with *our* own name, and even come to like it–because it's our name, it's part of us. For this book, I had thought to assume the nom de plume of B.G. Cole, but when it came time to actually see my name in print, I went with "Brad"—a likeable contraction of the stiff "Bradford"—but kept the "Colegate." "Cole" seemed like chopping a limb off the family tree.

We all have a right to be addressed as we wish, but sometimes communicating that wish can be difficult. Any "Charles" who is unwillingly reduced to "Chuck" can attest to that. For some, it's such an emotionally charged point that they suffer in silence rather than risk showing their anger. If you're someone with this problem simply practice saying "Please call me ____," until it's easy to say.

Physicians have earned the title "Doctor" through many difficult years of study and training, and view being as addressed as "Doctor ____" as a simple recognition of that fact, not as a snobbish title that separates them from the masses. Some patients may feel "Doctor" is too formal and distancing, while others subconsciously feel protected by the 'magical' power the word invokes. Since it's important for you to feel at ease with your physician to establish a good rapport, make sure you're addressing one another in a way that's comfortable for you both.

- *Do* tell your physician how you'd like to be addressed: "Bob," "Robert," or "Mr. Holcombe."

- *Do* ask if it's okay to call your physician by her first name, if you're more comfortable with that. Most physicians won't mind–they may even prefer it.

- *Do* expect that your doctor may ask you how you like to be called, especially if you're going to be a long-term patient that she'll be seeing–and addressing–many times.

- *Don't* call your doctor just "doc." (That sounds like something that belongs in a cartoon!)

The White Glove Patient

Mrs. Lucinda Cray had seen a lot of changes in her 71 years of living, and she herself had changed a lot, but one thing she wasn't about to give up was wearing her white gloves when out in public. She was aware that people thought it looked snobbish and peculiar, but she wasn't a snob–it was just that all those naked, sweaty hands embracing each other in the social ritual of handshaking seemed to her to be highly uncivilized. Besides, she hated looking down at all those liver spots on the back of her hands. Thank goodness she didn't have to look at her own face except when she was putting on her make-up in the morning. If she looked even half as old as her best friend of 50 years, Mayvis Johnson, she'd rather not be reminded of it.

She had dozens of pairs of gloves, and it amazed her how frequently she had to change them. No matter how careful she was, they never stayed clean more than a day. It was such a dirty world. Now here she was in Dr. Todd Peterson's office with time on her hands, and dust on her fingers. While waiting for him to come in and give her a refill for her thyroid medicine, she'd run her right index finger along the back of her chair and come away with the tip covered in gray fuzz.

"Don't you ever clean in here?" she asked abruptly as her doctor entered the room, wagging her incriminatingly dusty finger at him.

Dr. Peterson's cheeks flushed red. "Well, yes, of course. I mean, the office staff cleans the rooms after every patient, and then more thoroughly as needed."

"I'd say it needs it now," she declared. "You'd think a doctor's office, of all places, would be clean."

If you look hard enough, dust and germs are everywhere in the environment, including your doctor's office. Unless you happen to be allergic to dust, it's not a health hazard, and there's no cause for alarm if you see some in the office. Blood and bodily secretions, however, are another matter; there are strict guidelines that must be followed for dealing with those. When it comes to surgical procedures, materials and equipment should be not only clean but also sterile. In reality, you and your physician, not the physical environment, are the greatest biohazards in the office. So not only will your physician wash his hands before and/or after his encounter with you, but so should you. And save the white gloves for the opera.

- *Do* expect your physician's office to be tidy, but not spotless.

- *Do* expect surgical supplies and equipment to be sterilized.

- *Don't* handle something that looks like it may be contaminated with bodily fluids, but do let the physician or office staff know about it.

- *Do* wash your hands after you leave the office, to reduce the chance of picking up or transmitting an infection.

Patients Who Don't Like Doctors

Dick Stein looked like he was seeing a ghost rather than his new physician. As the white-clad image of Dr. Lionel Hemingway appeared before his eyes, Mr. Stein turned pale, and drops of sweat gathered at his brow. As he took Dick's clammy hand in greeting, the physician said, "I'd ask you how you're feeling, but it's obvious you're not feeling very well today."

"Oh, I'm all right," he replied. "I'm just here for a refill on my nasal spray. But I don't like doctors, and I don't like needles."

"Well, I'm glad you don't like needles, but I hope you'll eventually look on me as your ally."

"Don't count on it."

Dr. Hemingway flashed a forced smile. "Let's just go ahead and get you your refill and you can be on your way."

They were both in such a hurry to see the last of one another that Mr. Stein failed to mention the abdominal pains he'd been having lately while playing tennis, and Dr. Hemingway certainly didn't encourage further communication. Two weeks later, when Mr. Stein was hospitalized with a dissecting abdominal aneurysm, he found out he not only didn't like doctors— he didn't like surgery or hospitals either.

Most people don't like to go to the doctor's office, and those who actually *do* like it are not only in the minority but may have a problem: hypochondriasis. No one likes pain (needles), expense (X-rays), wasted time (the waiting room), and most of all, fear–the fear that *something is really wrong with you*. Previous unhappy experiences in the office or hospital often increase your anxiety and sense of dread and become a self-fulfilling prophecy that the visit will be something you "don't like."

A cheerfully appointed waiting room, a friendly staff, and a physician with a likeable and soothing manner go a long way towards making the encounter as pleasant as possible. We physicians know there are other places you'd rather be–we just don't want to hear about it.

- *Do* remember that doctors don't like your disease either; they like helping you get better.
- *Don't* tell you doctor that you "don't like doctors"; if you've had bad experiences in the past, try not to generalize.

- *Do* focus your negative feelings on your illness rather than those who are trying to help you.

- *Do* remember that just as you'd rather be elsewhere than a doctor's office, so would your physician rather be "gone fishing" (or golfing, or gardening, or sailing).

The Self-Destructing Patient

"I've got one whopping case of heartburn, doc," said Jasper Maycomb as he leaned forward on the examining table.

"Are you drinking again, Jasper?" asked Dr. Laura Bradbury, his physician, who had followed his successes and relapses with various drug rehab programs for the past twenty years.

"Not for the last two days. It feels like my stomach's on fire if I drink anything, even beer. I need some of that acid-blocking medication you gave me a few months ago."

"So you can get better, or so you can resume drinking?" Her patient's hesitation gave her the answer. "I don't want to prescribe the medication unless you agree to enter rehab again," she told him.

"I promise," he said, holding up his right hand, Boy Scout-style. "That last program at Mt. Cedars was pretty good. They said I could just call them if I ever needed more help."

"Okay. I'll put you back on the medication, but I'll need to see you again next week."

She did see Jasper the next week: not in the office, but in the emergency room, where he was found to have a bleeding ulcer. (His stomach had been feeling so much better on the medication that he didn't think a quart of bourbon would hurt anything!)

Doctors like to help people get better and stay that way, so it's frustrating when patients do things that defeat their efforts. It's like digging a hole while someone else keeps shoveling dirt back into it.

Sometimes people think that they can continue to drink, smoke, and do drugs because modern medicine will always have a means to rescue them from the consequences of their behaviors. It's not true. If you keep swimming with sharks, we can throw you a lifeline time after time, but sooner or later–you're gonna get eaten.

- *Don't* use illegal drugs.
- *Don't* drink alcohol excessively (more than one or two drinks per day).
- *Don't* smoke at all.

- *Do* expect your physician to counsel you (or, perhaps from your point of view, "lecture" you) regarding the above, even when you come into the office for unrelated reasons.

- *Do* ask your physician for her help if you're trying to stop smoking, drinking, or using drugs.

"Special" Patients

Soprano Patrice Von Stade was an imposing figure on the stage. At 5' 10" and 186 pounds, she had a voice as big as the rest of her, and well-suited to her specialty of Wagnerian heroines. Brushing another woman aside, she stepped up to the reception desk at Dr. Frank Colter's office and said, "I need to see Dr. Colter immediately!"

"Is it an emergency?" queried the receptionist.

"Yes, it is. I'm getting a cold," Patrice replied, coldly.

Raising her eyebrows, the receptionist said, "I'm afraid that doesn't qualify as an emergency."

"For me it is. I'm opening tonight in *Tristan und Isolde* in Indianapolis."

"I see," the receptionist replied, yawning as she looked at the daily schedule. "You're in luck. We had a cancellation for 10:30. You can have that, but you'll have to wait your turn."

As she waited, Patrice could feel her throat getting tighter and tighter. By the time Dr. Colter saw her, her voice was–*horrors!*–a little hoarse.

"I need to nip this thing in the bud, doctor. I must be able to sing tonight."

"Well, it's probably a virus, and viruses don't care much for opera."

Ms. Von Stade didn't laugh. "I don't care what the cause is, I need to get rid of it. Do whatever you can."

"I doubt if it will help, but I'll put you on antibiotics, just in case it's bacterial. Other than that, take acetaminophen and plenty of fluids and lozenges and all the things I recommend for anybody with a cold."

"But doctor," she said, stiffening in her chair, "I'm not just anybody."

Death may be the great leveler, but so is its ally, Disease. We all get sick from time to time, no matter how wealthy, famous, or talented. Still, we all think of ourselves as special, and when we see our physicians we present ourselves as having special needs. The singer with a cold, the professor with plugged-up ears who's leaving on a plane for Europe, the bridesmaid with a weight problem who wants to lose 10 pounds two weeks before the wedding, all have a sense of urgency about their problems, and try to parlay this into receiving special treatment that other folks with the same condition might not receive. But it's still the same condition; a cold is a cold is a cold.

While the above is true for common problems, sometimes people develop unique problems related to their particular field of endeavor, and these can indeed require special treatment. For instance, a singer who develops vocal cord nodules needs to see an otolaryngologist. So sometimes we are special after all.

- *Do* realize that diseases are no respecters of persons.
- *Do* tell your doctor about your "special" circumstances, but,
- *Don't* expect it to necessarily make a difference in your diagnosis and treatment.

The Lawyer

At age 32, Gabriella Martinez had just become the youngest partner in the law firm of Hansen, Arles, & Martinez, specializing in contract law. If anyone could find a loophole to get a client off the hook, she could. And likewise, if the client was trying to enforce any clause of the agreement, Ms. Martinez was the one who could make it stick. It was natural for her to see the rest of her life in contractual terms: she had just completed a prenuptial agreement with her fiancé, and had no reason to believe her relationship with her doctor should offer any less of a guarantee.

So when she came to the office concerned about a recently-noted lump behind her left ear, she wanted everything spelled out in black and white.

"What exactly is it, doctor?" she asked.

"Feels like a sebaceous cyst," replied Dr. Sheila Casey, who had seen thousands of these in her career. "It's just a plugged-up oil gland–nothing to worry about."

"But are you certain?"

"Well, it feels typical: round and smooth, slightly compressible, and it's in a location where they typically occur."

"You're 100 percent sure?"

"Well, no. Nothing is 100 percent, unless we cut it out and have it looked at under the microscope. But I doubt that you'd want to go through all that."

"Maybe I do. After all, if you're wrong, I wouldn't want to have to sue you for malpractice."

"No," said Dr. Casey, shaking her head, "I wouldn't want that either."

Most lawyers are good patients and good people, and some of them I count as friends. Still, having them as patients can be a little intimidating.

Attorneys are trained to look for the hard terms, the details, and the promises or guarantees in a business interaction, and so tend to look for these things from their physicians. But physicians can't make any firm guarantees, since the practice of medicine is still as much an art as a science.

- *Don't* ask for a guaranteed outcome or effectiveness of treatment.
- *Do* expect the physician to explain what a reasonable or likely outcome would be.

- *Do* expect to be warned about common serious side effects or adverse outcomes.

- *Don't* expect to be warned about rare or minor side effects–that would take all day!

- *Do* discuss with your physician any frustrations or disappointments you have with your medical care.

The Queen of Extraneous Details

Dr. Sandy Thomason thought she was making a simple request about a simple problem. "Tell me about your cold," she had said.

Her patient, twenty-something Mary Ellen Bosch, was more than happy to oblige. Working as a dental hygienist, she knew details could be important, so she didn't want to leave anything out. "Well, it all started last Thursday when I sat out in the cold at my son's Little League game. It was only about 50 degrees that evening and I'd forgotten to bring my jacket. Can you believe how cold it is for May? And to top it all off, they lost the game! Anyhow, by the time I got home I was already feeling sick. So I took my temperature and it was normal, but it was just one of those little plastic strips you stick under your tongue, so I'm not sure how accurate it is. Then I started getting congested and coughing up all sorts of brown phlegm–really gross stuff, like I'm a smoker or something but I'm not, though sometimes I'm tempted to start just to help get some of this extra weight off. And my throat feels scratchy, kinda like it's just dry, but drinking fluids doesn't help, even though I've been downing herbal tea like crazy–I found this great new mango pineapple flavor that I just love. And so then I got nauseated, but I thought it was just the hot dog and coffee I ate at the ball game. I know I shouldn't have eaten them because of all the nitrites and caffeine, but one of the other mothers was selling them as a fund-raiser, plus I was hoping they might warm me up a little. But then I had a bowel movement and I felt better, so maybe I was just constipated. So I went to bed hoping it was some kind of 24-hour bug, but when I woke up the next day…"

Sherlock Holmes realized that even the most minor details may be the vital clues that crack a case. Your doctor acts as a medical detective every time she makes a diagnosis, but if there is too much clutter in the way, she may have difficulty seeing the underlying problem.

Give your doctor all the appropriate information about your illness. Granted, it can sometimes be difficult for you to decide what to tell her and what to leave out; the answer lies somewhere between responding to all her questions with monosyllables and giving a minute-by-minute unedited stream of everything you can remember. The right balance can vary with the particular illness and its severity. You don't need to describe a cold in as much detail as chest pain, for example; in discussing your chest pain, it may be important that it occurred while just sitting on the couch watching

TV (as opposed to while exercising), but it's not important what program was on when you got the pain. Still, when in doubt, don't leave it out!

- *Do* run through the story of your illness in your head *before* you see the physician, in order to clarify it and to get the sequence of events down.
- *Do* write things down and bring that information with you if you have trouble remembering it but feel it's important.
- *Do* respond to your physician's questions even if you think the answers are not relevant to your illness; what you think is important and what she thinks is important may be two different things.
- *Do* allow the physician to interrupt you with necessary questions or help you refocus your story if it's getting off track.

The Medical Student

Craig Hollowell had just begun his cardiology rotation at Grant Hospital, an exciting month in his medical education, filled with all sorts of life-threatening diseases and life-saving technologies. Just this morning, he had been on the team that had given TPA–a blood clot dissolving agent–to a woman who was having a heart attack, or "acute myocardial infarction," as he would now call it. The wonder drug had performed miraculously well, opening up the circulation to her heart before any significant damage had been done. The experience made him feel a rush of medical power–and a shudder of vulnerability, to see how the blockage of one tiny artery could potentially kill someone. As he reviewed his textbook on coronary artery disease that night, he felt suddenly more aware of his own heartbeat, and a certain heaviness in his chest. He went to bed, thinking rest would help, but couldn't fall asleep, afraid that he might never wake up again. The next morning, he appeared in Dr. Gerald Mackenzie's office—for the fifth time in the last seven months.

As the physician greeted his patient, he couldn't help but ask, "Well, Craig, what's the disease-of-the-month this time?"

"I've been having chest pressure, and thought I should get an ECG and a treadmill stress test to rule out coronary artery disease."

"Craig, you're 24 years old. How likely do you think it is that you have heart disease at your age?"

"Well, I know I'm probably overreacting, but it's not impossible that this is something serious. I keep reading about all these diseases, and somebody has to be getting them–and it could be me." He paused, then said, "Sorry to keep bugging you."

"No problem," Dr. MacKenzie replied with a laugh. "Someday you'll have patients who are just like you."

Medical school is the time that many young people come face-to-face with mortality. After dealing with death and disease all day long, they go home to read about those diseases, all alone until the wee hours of the morning. It's no wonder that they themselves develop the well-described "medical student syndrome," in which they fear they have contracted the conditions they're studying: heart disease on the cardiology rotation, brain tumors on the neurology rotation, skin cancer on dermatology, and so on. Overwhelmed with information, but lacking in experience, they find that "a little bit of knowledge is a dangerous thing."

- *Do* come in for evaluation if you're having symptoms. You're not invulnerable to illness and you really might be sick and not "just imagining it."
- *Don't* prescribe your own diagnostic evaluation and therapy. Your physician, who has at least a few more years of experience than you, is in the best position to do that, but,
- *Do* share your concerns about what you think is wrong and what you thought might be done about it.
- *Don't* ask the residents you're working with to spend two minutes examining you and treating you. That's not fair to either of you.
- *Don't* swipe sample medications from the drug representatives to self-treat without seeing a physician.
- *Do* follow up by phone or in the office if you're advised to do so, even if you think you've figured it all out by yourself in the meantime.
- *Don't* expect your physician to know all those minute statistical details about your suspected illness that you just gleaned from your textbooks and that may have no relevance to the day-to-day office practice of medicine.

The Physician

Dr. Brad Lee was late for his appointment with his dermatologist, Dr. Kelly Kantrowicz. A family physician, Dr. Lee had seen several extra patients with urgent problems that morning and so was running 45 minutes late. He was surprised and a little irritated when he finally showed up in Dr. Kantrowicz's office that she wasn't ready to see him. *"You'd think she'd know how valuable my time is,"* he thought.

Finally the dermatologist entered the room–without apologizing for her lateness. *"He should know what it's like,"* she thought.

"Hi, Brad!" she chirped.

"'Brad'? She doesn't know me that well," he thought. "Hello, Dr. Kantrowicz," he countered.

Then he told her about the scaly, red skin condition on his face that he'd been self-medicating with a cortisone cream for the past four years. It hadn't been responding well–worsening, as a matter of fact, to the point that some days his face looked as bad as a teenager's with raging acne. Even his own patients would ask from time to time what was wrong with his face, and he was starting to feel like a leper.

"I thought it was seborrhea," he explained, "since I've had trouble with that on my scalp ever since I was a kid. But it's not coming under control with what I've been using."

"That's because it's rosacea, not seborrhea," she said.

"Oh. Really. Are you sure?" asked Brad, not disbelieving her but feeling like an idiot.

"Yes. It's classic. The cortisone takes the red out temporarily, but doesn't stop the rosacea. I'll put you on some tetracycline capsules and metronidazole cream."

"Fine. I know tetracycline is cheap, but do you have some samples of the cream that I could use?"

"I do have samples, but I like to save those for my patients who don't have insurance. Your prescriptions will be probably be covered by your insurance."

"Alright. Oh, while I'm here, could you take off this little bump on the end of my nose? It seems to have gotten a bit bigger lately, and I'm not sure what it is."

Glancing at her watch before glancing at the spot he was pointing out, Dr. Kantrowicz said, "It would be better if you could come back for that another day, so we can schedule enough time–perhaps when you come in for your follow-up appointment."

"'Follow-up appointment?' I thought I'd just come back if it's not getting better."

Ignoring him, she said, "How about four weeks from now?"

"That's an awful long time if this thing on my nose happens to be cancerous. How about next week?"

"*How about never?*" thought the dermatologist.

Physicians ought to be ideal patients. Familiar with the terminology and technology of the profession as well as the office routine, you would think we would be timely, patient, courteous, and willing to do whatever our colleagues recommend. We ought to know the dangers of denial and self-diagnosis and so seek medical care at the appropriate time. We should be able and willing to pay promptly for our care.

But as the vignette illustrates (which, by the way, was based on my own case), physicians can be the worst patients of all. We fuss around treating ourselves with the wrong medications after having made the wrong diagnoses, and then seek help only when things are really messed up. We show up late–and then want to go to the head of the line. We have good insurance, but still want freebies–or "professional courtesy," as it's sometimes called. In short, we want special treatment.

After listing the various "problem patients" I've encountered, I thought it only fair to end with the physician, so you can see we're not exempt from judgment. Rather, we're like everybody else: flawed, needy, irritating, fascinating, wonderful–human.

- *Do* show up on time for your appointment.
- *Don't* expect your own difficult schedule to take precedence over that of the colleague you're consulting.
- *Do* consider a "first patient of the morning" appointment–before you've had a chance to start running late.
- *Don't* expect free care.
- *Do* heed your colleague's advice. After all, you're probably seeing a specialist who has more expertise in that area than you do!

TIME & MONEY

"I Have This Form For You To Fill Out"

Dr. Wilma Dickerson had just concluded her evaluation of Se-Oh Chan, a 43-year-old Chinese-American woman who was under treatment for hypertension. Having written the prescription for her medication (an ACE inhibitor), and having advised her to return in three months for a recheck, Dr. Dickerson was rising up from her chair to leave.

"Oh, doctor," said Mrs. Chan, "could you please fill out this form for my insurance company?"

Dr. Dickerson reluctantly took the piece of paper Mrs. Chan was holding out to her and glanced at it. The front side was for the patient's personal information, such as address and telephone number, while the back side was headed by the phrase "TO BE COMPLETED BY THE PHYSICIAN" with a litany of questions and blank spaces to be filled in: Illness or condition work-related? Will further treatment be necessary? And so on.

The doctor handed the form back to Mrs. Chan and said, "Jenny, our business manager, can help you with that. Just drop it off as you're leaving."

"But it says you're the one who is supposed to complete it, and see–there's a place for your signature."

"My office staff handles these things."

"It would only take you a minute. I don't want to have to come back for this."

"I'm sorry, but I need to spend my time seeing patients, not doing paperwork."

As the physician turned and left the room, Mrs. Chan could feel her previously well-controlled blood pressure rising.

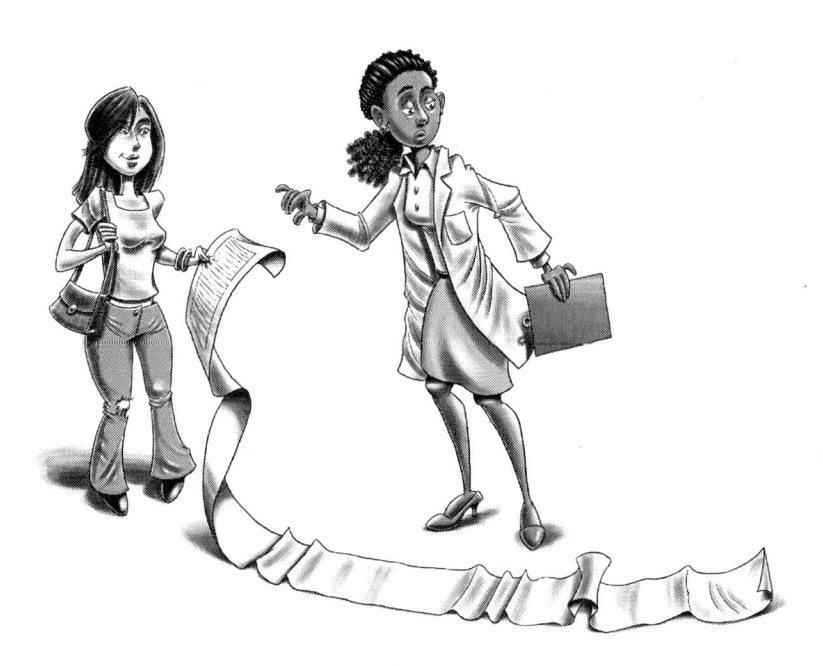

"I have this form for you to fill out."

Year by year, the paperwork involved in running a doctor's office has gotten more and more complicated, consuming more and more of the office staff's and physician's time. The staff member whose job depends on handling most of the billing and insurance claims may appreciate the paperwork, but the physician does not. I feel safe in saying that there's not a single physician in the entire country who enjoys filling out insurance forms; it's a necessary evil that the doctor tries to minimize and defers to her employees whenever possible.

Medical schools and residencies are now trying to educate their students and residents about the realities of medical business, office administration, and paperwork. But it certainly has nothing directly to do with the reason they entered training: to take care of patients.

- *Do* expect the office staff to assist you in completing the paperwork necessary for your insurance coverage.

- *Do* complete as much of your forms as you can yourself before approaching the office staff for help.

- *Don't* expect the physician to complete all your forms personally; she may forward them to her office staff.

- *Don't* expect the staff to drop everything else to fill out your forms while you wait.

Staff Members

Dr. Murray White's 36-year-old office nurse, Betty Koster, was congested, coughing, and feverish–like half the patients he'd been seeing that week. The wintertime spate of respiratory infections had left no openings in his office schedule, but he was "working in" additional sick patients. It was going to be a long day. So it was naturally a bit disconcerting when his nurse asked him, "Could you take a look at me, doctor? I've got a terribly itchy rash that's starting to spread."

"Well, as you know, I'm already running half-an-hour behind this morning. Maybe I could check you early this afternoon."

"How about over your lunch break?"

"I've got a lot of phone calls I need to make then."

"Maybe you could just give me some of those antihistamine samples the drug rep left us."

"No, I can't do that. If you're going to be treated, you're going to be examined, just like anyone else."

"Oh, for gosh sakes! I'm not just any old patient. I'm your nurse."

So Dr. White stopped what he was doing, checked her over, and diagnosed her as having hives from an allergic reaction to her new enzyme-based laundry detergent. Although this only took a few minutes, it put him further behind–and put a noticeable strain on his working relationship with his nurse. By the end of the day, they were both "itching" to get away from one another and go home.

Staff members in any office enjoy having "perks" uniquely related to their jobs. Clothing store salespeople enjoy discounts on their own merchandise; carpet installers take home remnants of rugs; workers at the license bureau never have to stand in line to wait for their own driver's licenses. So it's perfectly natural for medical office workers to feel they should have special access to medical care.

But this creates a number of problems. If care is provided without charge, it means the physician is losing time and an appointment slot that could have been used for a paying patient. Frequently, staff (who may have prescription drug coverage) want to be given the free samples of medications from pharmaceutical companies, which are often reserved for patients without insurance who might not otherwise be able to afford medication. Staff members often request their physicians to cut corners in order to save on costs–such as not ordering lab tests to help in diagnosis.

And if something goes wrong or the staff member is not responding well to treatment, the resultant tension can ruin their ability to work together.

- *Do* consider having your own private physician even if care in the office is provided free of charge.
- *Do* discuss with your employer (at the time you are hired) what his policy is regarding providing care for employees–and respect it.
- *Don't* expect your physician to cut corners that might handicap him in providing you with the best care.
- *Do* at least have your own gynecologist.
- *Do* follow your physician's advice—even if it's free. (We often don't value that which is free as highly as things we have to pay for.)
- *Don't* use your experience in the office to self-diagnose and self-treat.

"I Don't Have Time To Be Sick"

David Moore was a busy man. The 28-year-old industrial arts teacher was attending law school in the evenings, as well as trying to fulfill his duties as a husband and father. But with the sudden onset of nausea, cramps, and diarrhea, he was unable to get anything done. He called his doctor's office and was relieved to hear they could squeeze him into the morning schedule. If he got out by noon, the day might not be entirely wasted.

As he examined David, Dr. Jeff Minor noticed his patient repeatedly glancing at his wristwatch, but he continued to do a careful, methodical evaluation. Then he gave his diagnosis: "I think it's a viral gastroenteritis. I'll give you something to control the symptoms, but it's not a cure. This should run its course in a few days."

David was incredulous. "A few days! I can't afford to feel like this for 'a few days.' Doctor, I don't have time to be sick!"

"The virus doesn't care about that."

"Well, and neither do you, from the sound of it. And I don't have time for this crap," he said as he stomped out of the room.

The microbes that invade your body, the illnesses that overcome you, and the injuries that disable you are mindless, uncaring entities that don't realize you have better things to do and are on a timetable.

Your physician cares about you and wants you to get well as soon as possible, but he can only do so much to hurry things along. Even with a cast on, broken bones require a few weeks to heal; even with antibiotics, bacterial infections take a few days to resolve. This is not much solace for an actor getting ready to go on stage, or a businessman gearing up for a major presentation, or a college student facing a final exam the following day–but it's the way Nature works, and at best, a physician is Nature's assistant.

- *Do* let your physician know about the deadlines you're facing.
- *Do* expect him to be sympathetic, but
- *Don't* expect him to be able to perform a miracle to help you meet your deadline.

- *Do* realize that getting better requires the proper amount of time as well as the proper treatment.

"Just Phone It In"

Dr. Sheryl Fein's nurse looked exasperated. "It's Geraldine Johnson on the phone for you. I tried to tell her she needs to come in for an appointment, but she insists on speaking with you."

Sighing, Dr. Fein said, "You know what she's like. Better put her through."

"Thanks so much for taking my call," began Mrs. Johnson. "It's just a little problem and I'm sure it's something you can handle over the phone, and so that'll save you the bother of having to see me in the office."

"*And save you the price of an office visit,*" thought Dr. Fein, but said, "And what is this 'little problem?'"

"Well, I've been having some stomach cramping just like last year when I had that ruptured ovarian cyst, and I wondered if you could call in some pain medication for me."

"No, I don't think that's a good idea. Abdominal pain can come from so many different causes–it could be something else this time."

"But I just don't have time to come in right now. My daughter's getting married this Saturday and we've got a million things to do. The pain's usually not bad during the day and I take Tylenol for it, but I need something stronger at night so I can sleep. I'm not running a fever or throwing up or anything else. I *know* it's the same thing as before." Then she played her trump card. "I've been your patient for nearly 15 years now, Dr. Fein. You know you can trust me to come in if I don't get better."

So the patient got her pain medicine, but she didn't get better–she got much worse, so bad that she called 911 in the middle of the night, and was rushed to the hospital for emergency surgery. As it turned out, her "ovarian cyst" was an ectopic pregnancy.

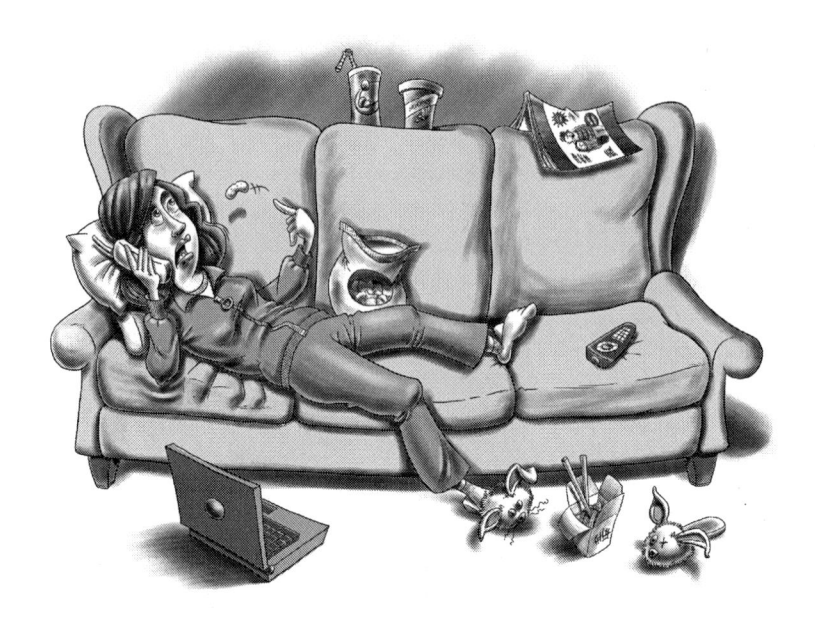

The telephone is a wonderful adjunct to your relationship with your doctor: it's a good way to check on test results, to inform the doctor about side effects of medication, and to get in touch in case of an emergency. But it's not a replacement for a face-to-face encounter. The sound of a telephone can communicate only so much information; it can't show the doctor what color your throat is or how tender your elbow is.

In order to properly diagnose a problem, a physician needs information not only from what you tell her, but from what she can see, hear, and feel (and rarely, smell!) on the physical exam. So when she (or her nurse) tells you she needs to see you in the office to take care of your problem, it isn't just because she wants to make money from you (although that *is* how she earns her living!)

- *Do* telephone your doctor to schedule an appointment, check on test results, and inform the doctor of any significant side effects of treatments.
- *Do* call 911 first instead of the doctor's office if you're experiencing a true emergency (hemorrhaging, suspected heart attack, stroke).

- *Do* come in to the office for an exam if the office nurse advises you to do so.

- *Don't* expect your doctor to diagnose and treat your problem over the phone.

- *Do* call to ask if routine refills of medications you take regularly can be phoned in–perhaps just to give you enough to get you through until you can come to the office for a check-up.

The Impatient Patient

Daniel Woodbury had already thumbed through the old copies of *Sports Illustrated*, *Field & Stream*, and *Newsweek* in Dr. Grant Harding's waiting room, leaving only the "women's" magazines to peruse. He was considering reading an article about flower arranging by Martha Stewart, when he was rescued by the voice of the office nurse calling "Mr. Woodbury–you're next!"

Even after he was seated in the exam room and had his vital signs taken by the nurse, there was still a wait of another 15 minutes before Dr. Harding appeared. He saw a white coat flash by the open door a few times before the doctor rushed into his room and said a breathless "Good morning!"

"'Good morning?'" said Mr. Woodbury with a pinched mouth, looking like a schoolteacher chiding a pupil for giving the wrong answer. "Another 10 minutes and it would be 'good afternoon.'"

"Sorry I'm running so far behind."

Mr. Woodbury was not to be placated by a mere apology. "I had an appointment for 10:45 and here it is 11:51 already. I'm a busy man too, you know. My time is just as valuable as yours."

"Yes, of course, you're right. It's just that I had to see a patient on an emergency basis at the hospital this morning and then I had several urgent patients added to my office schedule, and…"

"Maybe you need to take those possibilities into account ahead of time. In my dry cleaning business, I know how many pieces I can handle each day, and I know when they'll be ready for people to pick up. I don't make promises I can't keep."

"Neither do I. An appointment time is an estimate, not an iron-clad guarantee."

"Be that as it may, I've lost an extra hour of business due to your being late, and time is money. I ought to send you a bill for an hour of my time."

"Fine. Don't expect to be paid."

"And don't expect to have me as a patient ever again." With that, he walked past the doctor and out of the office.

Dr. Harding never did find out what the man's problem was–other than a lack of patience.

Everybody's in a hurry nowadays; everybody hates to wait. I hate standing in line for a movie ticket, or waiting at the fast-food counter for my cheeseburger and fries (yes, I know it's junk food), and I even hate waiting to see my physician. But a physician's office is not a factory, producing a uniform product exactly every ten minutes. Patients have varying needs and unpredictable problems that defy fitting into a rigid schedule; the physician needs to be flexible with his time–and so do you.

- *Do* realize that there's no way to predict ahead of time exactly how long an evaluation or appointment will take.

- *Do* realize that the doctor may be running late because the *previous patients* arrived late.

- *Do* arrive early or on time for your appointment even though you "know" you'll end up waiting–the physician may happen to be running on time that day!

- *Do* realize that emergencies often disrupt a doctor's schedule, and some day that emergency may be yours.

- *Do* take the other patients who are still waiting into consideration when you start thinking of additional problems to ask the doctor "as long as I'm here."

- *Do* realize that if your appointment is at 9:15 and the next one is at 9:30, you're not going to have a full 15 minutes of "face time" with the physician even if he's running on time. He'll also need time to document the visit in the chart (symptoms, findings, diagnosis, and treatment) and will need to squeeze in phone calls and paperwork between patients.

- *Do* let the staff know if you have a very urgent matter to attend to and the doctor is running late–they might be able to squeeze you in earlier–but try not to schedule important events too close to your appointment time.

- *Do* consider finding another physician if he's always running far behind and he makes no apology for it and the wait upsets you. Good luck!

The Laundry List

It was 10:30 a.m. and already Dr. Jake Hathaway was running 20 minutes behind schedule. He'd gotten to the office on time–10 minutes early, as a matter of fact–after making rounds on his hospitalized patients. But today it seemed as if all the patients had multiple or complex problems, and while he was doing his best to accommodate them, it was getting frustrating trying to catch up. So he was glad to see that the next patient, Mary Dugan, was listed by the nurse as having only "refill of acne medicine"–*that* should give him a few extra minutes.

"Good morning, Mrs. Dugan," he said. "Casey wrote down here that you're in for a refill of your tetracycline. Is that correct?"

"Yes," replied the red-haired high school Spanish teacher, "but I've got a few other things that I'd like you to check while I'm here. I wrote them all down so I wouldn't forget anything."

As she handed him the 8 x 11 piece of paper half-filled with writing, Dr. Hathaway could feel himself grinding his teeth. "I'm afraid I won't be able to address all these problems today, but I'll be happy to have Jennifer schedule you some additional time."

"I've been waiting here half an hour and you want me to come back again so you don't have to spend a few extra minutes with me?"

Dr. Hathaway sighed and looked at the piece of paper. "Well, let me see what I can do." It looked like it would be another five-minute lunch "hour" again that day.

People often wonder why physicians seem to be habitually behind schedule, and this type of patient is perhaps the biggest single factor. When a doctor has 15 minutes allotted to evaluate and treat the problem for which a patient has scheduled, it's nearly impossible to fit in one additional problem (let alone two or three) which may be even more complex than the original problem. There's simply no way to manufacture extra time out of thin air.

There are many reasons why patients mention additional problems for which they were not scheduled: they may have just thought of them while they were in the office; they may have mentioned the extra problems to the receptionist, who failed to schedule extra time; or they may be trying to get a "two-for-one special"–treatment of more than one problem for the price of one office visit. Whatever the reason, bringing in a "laundry list" of unscheduled problems is unfair to your physician, to the next patient on his schedule, and ultimately to *you*. If he's trying to squeeze several problems into one visit, he will probably rush, possibly be irritated, and certainly not give each problem the attention it deserves.

- *Do* tell the receptionist, when you call to schedule your appointment, if you have more than one problem.

- *Do* tell your physician about additional problems you "just happen to think of" when you're in the office, but try to do so at the beginning of the visit.

- *Don't* expect that the physician will necessarily be able to treat all your problems during one visit.

- *Do* make additional appointments if advised to do so for your extra problems.

The Deadbeat

Clara Trowbridge was irate, and Ben Sands, the business manager of Dr. Cynthia Waites' office, was unlucky enough to be on the receiving end of her phone call.

"Will you please stop sending me those bills!" shouted Clara. "I've told you before and I'm telling you now, I'm not going to pay them!"

"But you were seen and treated by Dr. Waites for your illness, so of course we expect payment."

"I've been trying to explain to you that I got nothing out of that visit. I came to her with a terrible headache, and two days later I had to see a different doctor for the same headache and I finally got some medicine that cleared it right up."

"Nevertheless, she spent her time dealing with you, and that's what she charges for: her time."

"Well, when I pay for something, I expect to get something back out of it, so don't hold your breath waiting for my money!" she said as she slammed down the phone.

The account was turned over to a collections agency, which was successful in recovering the payment due—and probably not as polite as Mr. Sands.

Physicians enter the field of medicine for many different reasons: because of the satisfaction involved in helping people, because of the intellectual challenges, because of the feeling of power and energy and sense of meaning they derive from what they do–and because of the money. Like anybody else, they have to earn a living, and the only way to do it is to charge for their services. But contrary to popular belief, greed is not the primary motivation for most physicians.

Physicians' relatively high incomes result from a number of factors. The typical physician attends high school, followed by four years of college, followed by four years of medical school, followed by at least three years of specialty training. What you're paying the physician hardly goes right into her pocket; the office overhead (staff salaries, rent, utilities, equipment, supplies, and malpractice insurance) typically consumes more than half the gross income of the practice. She can't afford to treat patients for free any more than a restaurant can give away free food. And please pay as promptly as possible; after all, you don't wait three months before paying for that steak dinner, do you?

- *Do* realize that a physician charges for her time, not for a specific result.

- *Do* realize that the expense of a visit involves paying for the highly specialized skills of a person who has undergone many years of difficult training.

- *Do* let your physician know if you're having trouble paying your bill. She or her office manager can help you arrange payments and perhaps even write off part of it if you have a low income.

- *Do* expect to pay more if your problems are more complex or require more time or testing.

The Referral Refuser

Martin Van Amman, a retired farmer, had been living in his condo in Virginia Beach for nearly 10 years, but he was still suffering the effects of all those years of sowing, tending, and harvesting fields of corn in the Indiana sun. He had a recurring crop of actinic keratoses (precancerous lesions) on his face for which he was under treatment. Even worse, he'd previously had a malignant melanoma: a tiny bleeding black pearl of death which Dr. Peter Brooks had discovered during a routine exam and had excised before it metastasized.

Now Martin had a nodule growing at the left side of his nose. It didn't worry him much at first. After all, it wasn't brown or black, so he doubted it was another melanoma. He just kept an eye on it for a few months, but once it had grown to the size of a pea, he knew he'd better see the doctor.

"Looks like a basal cell carcinoma," said Dr. Brooks. After seeing his patient's concern, he quickly added, "It's not nearly as serious as a melanoma, since basal cell cancers almost never metastasize. Still, it can keep growing and destroy your nose, so you've got to have it removed."

"Well, then, go ahead and take it off. Can you do it today?"

"Oh, I'm afraid this is something which exceeds my expertise. I'll need to send you to a specialist."

"But you took off that other cancer."

"Yes, and it was a lot smaller and in a different location. For this one, you need someone who can perform a special type of surgery called Mohs' surgery."

"So I'll have to make another appointment and drive across town to some specialist for something you ought to be able to do right here. And I thought you were such a good doctor."

Bristling, Dr. Brooks defended himself. "I am a good doctor. That's why I want to send you to someone else. If I tried to remove that nodule, I'd be an idiot, not a good doctor."

Mr. Van Amman looked like he wasn't sure which one of those two possibilities was standing in front of him.

Physicians are trained in depth in a wide variety of subjects. But the amount of available knowledge is enormous–so enormous that no one individual can possibly absorb it all, unlike in centuries past when a physician was often a "Renaissance man," knowledgeable about all aspects of science, art, literature, philosophy, and religion.

Medical specialists nowadays focus on a certain, more narrow field, because they enjoy that particular type of practice–and because they enjoy *not* having to deal with the other areas. Ophthalmologists never have to evaluate people for diarrhea, orthopedists don't treat patients for depression, geriatricians don't have to examine crying 2-year-olds, and neurologists never have to worry about delivering a baby (except perhaps in an emergency on an airplane flight!)

So-called "generalists"–family physicians, pediatricians, and internists-can take care of perhaps 95% of your needs, but they can't do everything. Rather than expecting your physician to know and do everything, seek to find a doctor who knows his limits, who "knows what he does not know." Someone who acts as if he knows everything is not doing you any favors–but may do you harm.

- *Don't* expect your doctor to know and do everything.
- *Do* expect to be referred to a specialist from time to time.
- *Do* realize that a doctor who admits he doesn't know the answer to something is showing his honesty, not his ignorance.
- *Do* expect your doctor to have some plan as to how to proceed further if he doesn't know something, even if it's only to refer you to a specialist on the grounds that "two heads are better than one."

"Call Me"

Carrie Cordray was about to hit the big 3-0, and she was starting to worry about a lot of things–like whether she should marry her boyfriend of two years and perhaps start saving a little money instead of blowing it every payday. And maybe she should be more careful about her health; after all, if you can turn 30, she thought, you can hit 40, and even someday get *really* old. So she resolved to stop smoking, the one vice she had allowed herself because she'd never imagined reaching an age where the effects of smoking would be a concern.

Dr. Sheila Sommersby was happy to hear of Carrie's request to help her stop smoking. "That's great! That's the best thing you can do for yourself. And happy birthday, by the way."

"Thanks a lot," said Carrie grumpily.

"While you're here, I think we should also check your cholesterol. You've got a strong family history of heart disease, and cholesterol could be a factor."

"Fine, go ahead and check anything you think ought to be checked. You can just call me at my work number with the results."

"Well, I'll need to see you back in a couple weeks to see how you're doing with the nicotine patch. We'll go over the results then."

"But I really don't want to have to wait two weeks for the results."

"It's not anything urgent. High cholesterol takes decades to kill you."

"But the suspense of not knowing will worry me. Look, it's *my* blood and *my* test, so why can't I get the results when I want to?"

"Fine. Call the office two days from now, and the nurse can tell you the results."

"Oh, the nurse. So *you* don't want to be bothered."

Sighing, Dr. Sommersby said, "Okay. Here's the deal. I'll make a special note on my calendar to call you with the results." The doctor was a non-smoker, but by the time the encounter was over, they *both* felt like having a cigarette.

The practice of medicine nowadays seems to require some kind of specialized testing on nearly every patient: throat cultures for sore throats, blood profiles for fatigue, X-rays for injuries. Most of these tests are an appropriate part of the evaluation, and we do a lot more office testing than we did 30 years ago because it's available, reliable, and (relative to hospital-based testing) cheap. Some of the testing, of course, is due to the practice of "defensive medicine," as when a doctor orders an X-ray for a sprained ankle even though she feels it's extremely unlikely to be broken–so that if, on the one-in-a-thousand chance it is broken, it won't go undetected and be a basis for a malpractice suit.

With so much testing being done, evaluating the results and discussing them with patients has become a major part of a physician's day. Certainly a patient is entitled to know her test results, but there are different levels of interaction with the physician that one can expect, depending on the test and the patient's problem. The results of a biopsy to rule out cancer, for example, demands some kind of personal contact between the physician and patient—preferably an office visit, but at least a phone call with the discussion recorded in the chart. A report of cancer that doesn't get followed up is frequently the basis for a malpractice suit. On the other hand, minor abnormalities that don't seem to be related to disease, such as a slight decrease in the uric acid on a blood profile, are often not even discussed with the patient. The communication of some results may be delegated to the nurse (such as normal Pap smear results), or the physician my advise you to call in and check with the office staff (such as throat culture results). If you do have phone contact with a physician regarding tests results, she'll want to keep it short and to the point–it's not a time to "chat." Anything more will require an office visit.

- *Do* follow your physician's advice about how to obtain your test results —whether to make a return visit, to make a phone call, or to await notice from the office.

- *Do* call the office if you haven't heard about your results after a reasonable period of time, as occasionally results may get "lost in the cracks."

- *Do* realize that abnormal test results may require further visits, and further testing.

- *Do* remember that when you're on the phone with the physician, it's usually unscheduled time, and she has other patients waiting.

- *Don't* ask the physician to leave crucial or confidential results (such as cancer or sexually transmitted disease tests) on your answering machine or voice mail. She'll want you to hear those results directly from her.

"Oh, By The Way, Doc…"

At 6' 4" and 240 pounds, Dan Cassavetes, a former lineman for the Ohio State Buckeyes, was still a formidable sight at the age of 44. Though his opponents hadn't been able to knock him down to size, they had managed to inflict an injury to his right knee cartilage, which had been repaired by arthroscopic surgery, but which nonetheless led to some early arthritic changes.

"That knee acting up on you again?" asked his internist, Dr. Cheryl Bradley.

"Yeah. It hurts like the dickens when I get up in the morning. I know I could just take over-the-counter ibuprofen, but if you write for the prescription-strength tablets, my insurance will cover it."

"Okay, but take it with food, and let me know if it starts to upset your stomach." She did a brief exam of his knee just to make sure nothing had changed since his last visit, then gave him the requested prescription, and with her hand on the doorknob, prepared to make her exit.

Dan cleared his throat loudly and said, "Oh, by the way, Dr. Hadley, I've been having this little pain in my chest since this morning. Not a pain really, but more of a pressure. I'm probably just being paranoid—my dad died of a heart attack when he was 50—but do you think I should get it checked while I'm here?"

Dr. Hadley gritted her teeth. "*I think you should have told me about it before now,*" she thought. "Yes. It may just be your medicine causing some heartburn, but I'm a little paranoid about these kinds of symptoms too. Let's do an electrocardiogram."

She expected a reassuringly normal tracing, but felt her own heart racing when she saw the ECG. "It's a good thing you caught me before I got away from you, Mr. Cassavetes. You're going to the hospital–your tracing shows you're having a heart attack."

The sight of their physicians leaving the room has a stimulating effect on some patients: they suddenly remember a form that needs to be filled out, or a question about their prescriptions, and especially, additional medical problems. It's like the sight of the highway sign you're passing that reads: "Last Rest Area for the Next 60 Miles"—suddenly you realize your bladder is full. And sometimes it's only as the physician is leaving that the patient works up his nerve to ask about the problem that really brought him in to the office in the first place.

Naturally, for the physician who thought she had your visit all neatly wrapped up and was ready to move on to the next patient, this can be very disconcerting. It's like putting dinner on the table and just as you're sitting down to eat, someone asks if you could make a salad, too. Your doctor will first assess how urgent the problem seems to be, and then perhaps have you reschedule if it doesn't require immediate attention.

- *Do* let your physician know the real reason for your visit, up front!
- *Do* let your physician know if you have more than one problem, and do it at the beginning of the visit, but,
- *Don't* expect it will necessarily be dealt with on the same visit.
- *Do* try to prioritize your problems if you have more than one, and let the physician know which is the most important for you to have treated that day.

The Powder Room Patient

Terri Fletcher was proud of herself. She had not merely made it to her doctor's office on time for her appointment, she was early. But she found out that arriving early doesn't always translate into being seen early, so she was sitting waiting her turn, reading the latest *People*, but wishing she had brought the novel she'd been reading. Every few minutes she'd look up at the receptionist, who returned a smile that said, "*No, we're not ready for you yet.*"

As she was reading, she was also gulping the large coffee that she'd brought from a fast-food drive-in on the way to the office. By the time she finished it, the caffeine was doing a number on her kidneys, so she slipped down the hall to "freshen up." She didn't hear when the receptionist called, "Terri Fletcher! The physician is ready to see you," and when there was no response, "Oh, well, the next patient is here. Mr. Dornan, come right in."

Patients often complain about waiting and waiting to see the physician, but sometimes the tables are turned and the physician is waiting to see the patient. While in the waiting room, patients get bored and start to be aware of other things they need to do: go "powder their noses," make a phone call to their own offices, or even run an errand down the street (promising to be "back in a minute").

If your turn to be seen occurs while you're otherwise occupied, the physician may elect to use this time by making phone calls or seeing the next patient, the one who scheduled *after* you.

- *Don't* go to the bathroom (or at least check with the receptionist) if it's getting near your appointment time.
- *Do* try not to urinate before seeing the doctor if you have a urinary problem, since he'll need to examine a specimen of it. (And if you're having diarrhea, he may even need some of that!)
- *Don't* bring a urine specimen to the office in a home container. It won't be sterile, and traces of other substances (even in a visibly clean container) may interfere with the analysis.
- *Do* bring a book or needlepoint or something to occupy you while waiting.

FAMILY TROUBLES

The Menace

Having just celebrated his second birthday, Ronnie Frank was at the stage when he was not only curious about everything, but also had the capability to explore and examine those curiosities. His mother, Leila, was glad–on his good days–that she had such a bright and active child, and–on his bad days–wondered how she had given birth to such a holy terror. At home, where the medicines and the alcohol and the cleaning agents were all in locked cabinets (after a near-disaster when she'd caught him sniffing the window cleaner), she felt she could strike the proper balance between controlling him and allowing him to express his creativity. Away from home, like today at her physician's office, was another matter.

Dr. Amanda Jennings had other worries, however. "Put the tuning fork down, Ronnie."

Fascinated by the pure, high-pitched whine of the instrument, he was banging it against various pieces of office furniture. The physician was busy looking into Leila's ears, or else she herself would have snatched the instrument away from the child.

"Oh, he's just playing," said Leila.

With her best smile, Dr. Jennings replied, "But these aren't toys." Then she took the tuning fork, which Ronnie gave up easily, too surprised to resist.

"Perhaps we could have one of the staff watch him while I examine you."

"He'll get upset if he's not with me."

"Ronnie, get down from there!" ordered Dr. Jennings.

But it was too late. The child had already climbed atop the black leather wheeled stool and was using it for a trampoline. Leila laughed at her child's exuberance until she saw the stool roll out from under him. Ronnie fell to the floor and began to cry.

"No serious damage," said Dr. Jennings as she scooped up the child and handed him over to his mother.

"Well, I hope so," said Leila. "If he's hurt, I hope your insurance covers accidents in the office."

"Yes, it does," said Dr. Jennings. *"But it doesn't cover me for strangling you,"* she thought.

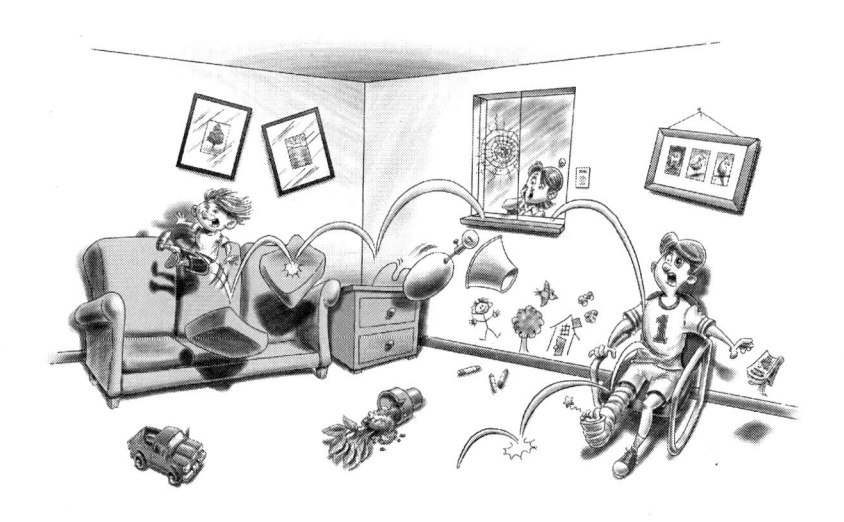

Children can be delightful, and children can be dreadful. Their unpredictability can be the source of great fun–or even tragedy. But unpredictable behavior does not mean *unmanageable*. Being a parent is a difficult, 24-hour-a-day job, and it certainly doesn't end when you're at the doctor's office. But if you consistently reinforce your child's good behavior in public (and private), the task should get easier with time—at least until they turn into teenagers.

- *Do* advise your child ahead of time how to behave in the office—not to touch the equipment, for example.
- *Do* physically restrain your child if he ignores your verbal instructions.
- *Don't* expect the office staff to be babysitters; they'll help when they can, but they have many other things to do.
- *Don't* expect toys and games to be provided by your physician, especially if you're the patient and you're seeing an internist or adult-care specialist. Bring your child's own toys along.
- *Do* consider hiring a sitter for your child the next time you have an appointment.

The Family Member

"Hi, Dad!"

"Andy! What's the matter?" Dr. Ted Gladdens was a bit alarmed to hear the voice of his eldest son greeting him. Ever since he started his intense MBA program, Andy only called if he needed something, and now his voice sounded weak and hoarse.

"I feel awful. I've got a fever of 102 and I'm tired and my throat hurts. I think it started after sitting out in the rain at the last football game."

"I *told* you to wear a raincoat." This slipped out before Dr. Gladdens realized how much he sounded like a nagging father.

"Okay, okay, you were right. Anyway, I was wondering what I should do to get rid of this infection ."

"Why don't you go see someone at an urgent care center?"

"I'm too busy. Besides, why should I do that when I've got a doctor for a father?"

Dr. Gladdens had always experienced mixed feelings about treating his own family members. What if he made the wrong diagnosis or something bad happened? But he knew he was as good a physician as anybody else, and besides, treating them himself was awfully convenient.

"It's probably just a bad cold virus. Take some of that cough medicine I sent along in your first-aid kit, and try to get more rest."

The next day he got another call, this time from Dr. Carrie Peterson, an emergency room physician at Crayton University Hospitals. "Your son Andrew was brought in last night by his roommate," she explained. "We admitted him with the diagnosis of strep throat complicated by dehydration." So instead of making a house call, Dr. Gladdens wound up making a hospital visit, and kicking himself for having tried to treat his son over the phone.

Refreshed by a few liters of IV fluids, Andy was feeling much better by the time his father arrived. Sitting up in bed, he smiled, then winked and said, "Next time, Dad, I'll talk to a *real* doctor."

Having a physician who is in the family treat you seems at first glance to have a number of advantages: no waiting room, no doctor's fee, and having him close by to monitor your condition. But it also means he may be tempted to jump to conclusions because he knows you so well, or he may ignore something bad because of denial–and then be wracked with a guilty conscience if something goes wrong. Doctors feel bad when any of our patients suffer ill effects from our treatments, so how much worse will we feel if they're our own family members?

- *Do* ask your physician-relatives for general medical advice.

- *Don't* ask them to diagnose and treat your specific ailments—or at least expect that you should be subjected to the same examination and testing that any patient would receive, and follow any treatment recommendations the same way.

- *Do* contact them about true medical emergencies, but call 911 first!

Dr. Mom

"My mother says I might have a sinus infection and I should come get an antibiotic," said Sylvia Chase, an 18-year-old college freshman away from home for the first time. "And I told her how tired I've been lately, and she says I'm not eating right and not getting enough vitamins, so she sent me a bottle of iron tablets and vitamin C and vitamin E."

"Are you a strict vegetarian?" asked Dr. Renata Manzoni, the middle-aged veteran physician at the college's student health center.

"No," Sylvia responded curtly.

"Then it's highly unlikely that you have a nutritional deficiency. There must be some other cause for your tiredness. Let me check you over."

On exam, Sylvia's lymph nodes ("glands") were markedly enlarged, prompting Dr. Manzoni to order a blood count to confirm her suspicion: infectious mononucleosis. "It's caused by the Epstein-Barr virus," she explained.

"Oh, no, not mono!" Sylvia groaned. "Final exams are coming up. What can we do to make the mono go away?"

"We can't make it go away, but we can treat your symptoms. Since it's a virus, antibiotics won't help. And those iron pills and vitamins won't do any good, either."

"Well, Mom isn't a doctor, but she was just trying to help."

"I know a way she can help. Why don't you go home this weekend and let her cook for you and do your laundry?"

Smiling, Sylvia agreed: "Now *that* sounds like a good prescription."

Mothers can be very wise people. Many of the problems I see every day in the office could probably be treated just as well by your mother. She'd say: if you're tired, you need more sleep and to eat better; if your foot hurts, put it up and take some ibuprofen; if you're stressed, do something relaxing and try to reduce your schedule. But it's not always that simple.

Mothers know us very intimately as individuals and are attuned to our moods and our state of health. They know when something is wrong but not necessarily *what* is wrong. So for your illnesses, let your mother cook the chicken soup, and let your doctor make the diagnosis.

- *Do* tell your mother about your illness and ask her advice.

- *Do* see your physician if your symptoms are severe or are not responding to home care.

The Silent Partner

Jim Casey was mad. After having been tested a few days ago for a discharge from his urethra, the young architect had just been diagnosed as having chlamydia, a sexually transmitted disease. "So that means my girlfriend's been sleeping around on me!" he said, spitting the words out.

"Not necessarily," Dr. Greg Geraldson replied. "You two have only been together for three months. Chlamydia can sometimes remain asymptomatic for several months, perhaps even a year or more on rare occasions. So maybe you got this from a previous partner."

"I don't think so," said Jim, barely calmer. "With my last girlfriend I used condoms all the time."

"But they're not foolproof. At any rate, the important thing is to tell your partner so she can be treated too."

"Hell, no!" he protested.

"You need to tell her so she can see her doctor and get some medication," insisted Dr. Geraldson. "Otherwise she's at risk for a pelvic infection and other complications."

"Her whole insides can rot out for all I care."

Dr. Geraldson couldn't help but think that the best prescription for his girlfriend would be to dump this guy ASAP.

The diagnosis of a sexually transmitted disease often leads to a dangerous game of pointing fingers: "You gave this to me!" "No, you got it first!" "I've been faithful. You must have been messing around on me." But let the *disease*, not your partner, be the enemy. You need to work together to conquer it or keep it under control.

Depending on the law in your state, you may also have a legal, as well as moral, responsibility to let your partner know of any diseases that may be transmissible by sexual contact. There have been lawsuits filed against partners (former partners) for "failure to inform."

Prevention should be the watchword. Get to know your partner and his or her sexual history; practice monogamy and use condoms, even during oral sex, since STD's can be carried in the throat. Treat your partner with the same respect and concern you expect for yourself.

If you refuse to tell your partner, you're putting your doctor in an ethical dilemma; he'd like to inform your partner, but the rule of confidentiality may prevent that, unless it's a disease that is reportable by law to your state's Department of Health. Your doctor's first obligation is to you, but he will not take kindly to your desire to wreak medical havoc on another human being.

- *Do* tell your partner about your diagnosis and treatment as soon as possible–in person, by phone, or by mail.
- *Don't* jump to conclusions about who gave what to whom.
- *Don't* use this as an opportunity to get revenge on your partner.
- *Don't* ask your physician to give you extra medicine for your partner without having her be seen in the office. She needs her own evaluation.

The Family Entourage

Dr. Jan Holcomb's exam rooms were quite commodious under most circumstances. At 12-by-12 feet square, there was room for an exam table, a sink, a small desk, a wheeled stool and two chairs. But today she could barely open the door to Exam Room 3, into which Susanna Pearlman and her family had already crowded. The elderly former art teacher had suffered a stroke three years ago which had left her with weakness on the left side of her body and difficulty speaking. Now, whenever she went somewhere–which wasn't very often–her strapping young grandson Keith would lift her into her wheelchair and push her, while her son and daughter-in-law supervised. Joe Pearlman, frightened by the sight of his enfeebled mother, mostly shrank into the corner while his wife Cynthia reluctantly took over Susanna's care. "Look out!" shouted Cynthia to her son. "The door's going to hit Grandma's foot!"

Keith pulled the wheelchair back away from the door and Dr. Holcomb crept into the room. The physician was greeted by a litany of complaints:

"Mom's got a sore on her toe."

"She's having trouble swallowing."

"Grandma's constipated."

Susanna was the only one who said nothing during the physical exam that followed.

"She doesn't say much anymore, doctor," explained Cynthia. "It's too hard for her to talk."

Or maybe she's given up trying to get a word in edgewise," thought Dr. Holcomb. After giving the family detailed instructions for the treatment of Susanna's problems, Dr. Holcomb tripped as she tried to ease her way toward the door, bumping into Cynthia and knocking her flat on her back. Although she remained silent, a lopsided smile crept across Susanna's face.

This time the difficulty wasn't with the patient, but her entourage. Family physicians like to see and treat the whole family–but not all at once. An exam room can get a little crowded with several family members jockeying for space, and the patient often gets lost in the shuffle.

There are numerous sound reasons for a family member to be in the room with a patient: a mother with her infant (either of whom could be the patient); a patient (such as Susanna) with a physical disability, who needs help with moving and/or speaking; or a patient who speaks a foreign language and needs an interpreter.

But, in most cases, minimizing the number of people in the room improves comfort and confidentiality, and clears the lines of communication for the physician to speak directly with the patient and develop the rapport that's needed for optimal diagnosis and treatment. A three-ring circus may be entertaining, but it's not the way to run a doctor's office.

If you are the patient:

- *Do* ask your family members to remain in the waiting room if there's no critical need for them to be present in the exam room.

If you are not the patient:

- *Do* allow the patient to tell her own medical history.
- *Do* try not to block the physician's path.
- *Do* step out of the room, if asked to do so (at least temporarily) if there are confidential things to be discussed, or if a private part of the body is being examined.
- *Do* add your own information and observations about the patient's illness when requested to do so.

The Teenager's Warden

In her own mind, Heidi Tober was a young woman, and at age 16, she had already reached her full adult height of 5' 6". But in her mother's mind, she was still a child. So when Heidi asked her mother, Janice, if she could go to the doctor for a "check-up," Janice naturally assumed she would go along with her daughter, just as she'd done for all the baby check-ups, immunizations, and illnesses in the past. And when Dr. Meg Livingston's nurse called Heidi to come to the exam room, Janice got up and accompanied her frowning child.

After her preliminary greetings, Dr. Livingston said, "So Heidi, you're in for a 'check-up.' Is there anything special you'd like to discuss?"

"Uh, no. No," said Heidi, casting a glance at her mother. "I feel fine. I just thought it would be a good idea to come in, since it's been awhile." She played with a handful of her ash-blonde hair as she fidgeted on the exam table.

Dr. Livingston turned to Heidi's mother. "Mrs. Tober, I'd like you to step out of the room while I continue with the exam, if you don't mind."

"Well, I certainly do mind!" replied Janice. "My daughter has no secrets from me. Do you, honey?"

"Be that as it may," interrupted the doctor, "I think it will work out better if you just have a seat in the waiting room. I'll have my nurse come in if I need help."

As Janice stomped out of the room, she said, "I'm sure you'll let me be involved when it comes time to pay for this."

Turning to her visibly more relaxed patient, Dr. Livingston said, "Well now, I'll ask you again: is there anything special you'd like to discuss?"

"Yes!" she said, and then reddened a bit. "I've got a boyfriend now, and I think I'd like to be on birth control pills."

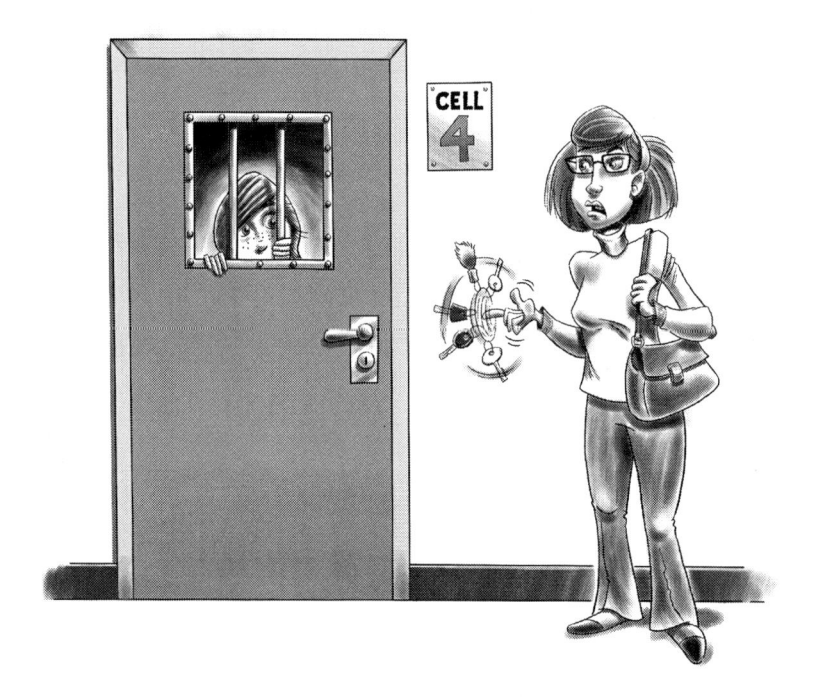

"You'll get out when you're 18, young lady."

A teenager has a right to privacy–even from her own parents. This applies not only to her room in the home, but the doctor's office as well. There are many issues a teenager may need to discuss with a physician that she may not wish to discuss with her parents: sexuality issues, drug use—even problems she's having with her parents. While a teenager may not mind having a parent in the room during an exam for a sore throat, she may be inhibited from bringing up other issues or answering questions honestly. Aside from any confidentiality matters, the teenager prefers to be treated as a young adult, without Mommy or Daddy hovering nearby.

The physician will encourage the patient to discuss important issues, like birth control, with her parents. In some cases, such as a suicidally depressed young person, the physician will seek to actively involve the parents. So it's not a conspiracy to exclude the parent, but an attempt to give the teenager an optimal environment for health care–the same thing her parents want for themselves.

- *Do* let your teenager see the physician unaccompanied, at least for part of the visit.

- *Do* leave the room if asked to do so by either the physician or your teenager.

- *Do* encourage your teenager to talk to the doctor about things they feel uncomfortable talking to you about.

- *Do* schedule your teenager for periodic health checks.

THE SEEKERS

The Siren

Kimberly Rose couldn't understand people who say they "hate to go to the doctor." She loved to go to the doctor, specifically, Dr. Jake Masterson, the tall, dark family physician who'd been taking care of her since she was a baby. He hadn't seemed to grow older as she did, just better looking. From time to time she fantasized about him, and lately, after his wife had died of breast cancer, she was thinking of him even more. He was always so friendly, giving her such a warm smile, that she felt special in his presence and felt certain there was something special between them— something more than the usual doctor-patient relationship.

She had come to him today complaining of palpitations. As he listened to her heart, with nothing but her red lace bra and a stethoscope between them, she blurted out, "Would you like to go out with me sometime?"

His icy response shocked her. "No. I never date patients." And then he gave her his diagnosis and treatment recommendations.

After he left, Kimberly put her clothes back on and never gave him the chance to see her naked again, professionally *or* socially.

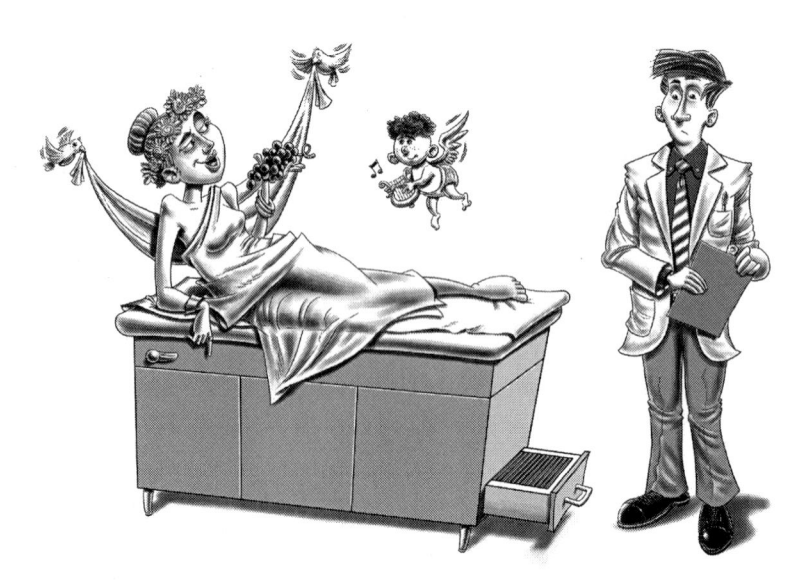

"I'm ready for my exam now, doctor!"

The doctor-patient relationship is a very intimate one. Your physician sees parts of your body that no one besides your spouse sees, and hears private details of your life that even your spouse may not know. Developing an attraction to your caregiver is a not uncommon phenomenon and is known as "transference." Sometimes the caregiver also develops an attraction, known as "counter-transference."

There have occasionally been instances where a physician has used his relationship and power over a patient to initiate a sexual relationship, which is unethical. But it also has happened that patients make advances toward their physicians, which is equally unethical. Being human–and there being only so many fish in the sea–there may occasionally be instances in which a romantic attraction may develop which both parties wish to pursue. It is recommended by some authorities that in such situations, the professional relationship be terminated and a "cooling off period" be observed before pursuing the romantic relationship. Things may look a lot different after six months of thinking it over.

- *Do* request a nurse or assistant as a chaperone if you feel uncomfortable being alone with the physician.

- *Do* expect the physician will likely have an assistant present during pelvic and breast exams, and, depending on the circumstances, rectal and male genital exams as well.

- *Don't* mistake the intimacy of being examined for a sexual encounter.

- *Don't* expect that seeing and touching you is a sexual thrill for the physician–it's just part of the job.

The Vitamin Junkie

At 5' 10" and 185 very muscular pounds, with a 29-inch waist, 33-year-old Franklin Reynolds looked like the perfect specimen of health and manhood. But today he was in the Clark County Emergency Room complaining to the doctor on duty: "I've been having bad headaches lately, and I'm starting to get worried about them."

As part of the history, Dr. Susan Willoughby inquired if Franklin was taking any medications.

"Just vitamins," he replied.

"Oh? And what vitamins specifically?"

"Some of everything: vitamin C, 1000 milligrams a day to keep from catching colds; a vitamin B complex pill; vitamin E, 1000 units twice a day; beta-carotene and a multivitamin with minerals, just in case I'm missing something. Oh, and I just started taking melatonin at bedtime. Plus I take a protein powder drink every day."

"That's a lot of supplements. Is it because you're a vegetarian?"

"No, I'm not a vegetarian. I lift weights; my body needs meat."

"Your dose of vitamin E sounds awfully high. Why so much?"

"Well, it's an antioxidant, and I'm not getting any younger, so I figure if a little is good, more is better."

"Does your multivitamin have vitamin E in it, too?"

"Sure does–400 units."

"So that means you're taking 2,400 units per day. Vitamin E is fat-soluble, so it can be stored by the body–meaning you can actually take too much of it and it can then cause symptoms like headaches. There are many different causes of headaches, but I think you'd better stop your extra vitamin E and just stick with the multivitamin."

"Okay, but can I take an extra melatonin then instead?"

Vitamins and other nutritional supplements are a matter of some controversy in the medical community. Some physicians take the view that "all they do is help you make very expensive urine." Others, like the Nobel Prize-winning Dr. Linus Pauling, who espoused vitamin C for preventing the common cold, believe that supplements can be helpful. Most Americans get plenty of nutrients from their daily intake of normal foods; vitamins are also added to some of our foods, such as cereals. Vitamins that are taken in excess of our daily needs are usually eliminated by the body rather than stored; the exceptions are vitamins A, D, E, and K, the so-called fat-soluble vitamins, which if taken in large doses can lead to potentially toxic levels, with resultant symptoms like headaches and vomiting.

In our search for well-being, to prevent illness, forestall aging, and to feel good, many of us look for a magic potion, and vitamins hold that allure for many. Certainly a single, combination daily multivitamin and mineral tablet is not a bad idea, but anything beyond that may be "fool's gold."

- *Do* eat a balanced diet.
- *Do* take a multivitamin if you want.
- *Don't* take "megadoses" of vitamins without discussing it with your physician first.

The Drug Seeker

Dr. Robyn Johns greeted her new patient enthusiastically: "Good morning, Mr. Pope! Nice to meet you!"

Bruce Pope, on the other hand, wasn't as cheery. The 28-year-old man was cradling his right jaw in his hand, and did not extend it to greet the physician. "I'm in awful pain, doc. I've got a terrible toothache and my dentist is on vacation in Mexico until Monday."

"Have you tried contacting another dentist?" asked Dr. Johns.

"Well, no. I've been going to Dr. Mitchell for years, and I'd rather wait for him to get back. I think I'll be fine if I can just get some pain medication."

"Let me take a look at you first. I'm not a dentist but maybe I can get an idea of what's causing the pain."

Peering into his oral cavity, she could see no particular signs of disease. Nor did palpating the tissues with a gloved finger reveal the source of the problem. "Can you show me the place where you feel the pain?" she asked.

"It's kinda hard to say. My whole jaw just throbs."

"Have you tried taking ibuprofen?"

"Oh, I'm allergic to that, and aspirin and all that stuff."

"What about acetaminophen?"

"That's like taking a sugar pill. You know, the only thing that seems to work for me is Ultracodeine."

Dr. Johns paused and considered the situation. "I suppose I could write you a prescription for a few, just to get you through until Dr. Mitchell gets back."

"But they don't work for me unless I take double the dosage. I guess I have a high tolerance. And could you make it refillable? After all, the weekend's coming up, and I wouldn't want to bother you again if I need some more."

"I'm sorry, but I'm getting the impression that the Ultracodeine is more important to you than your toothache. I don't think I should prescribe it for you."

Bruce looked at her coldly and knew he had been beaten. "Well, if you're just going to make insinuations, I don't think I want you as a doctor," he said as he rose to his feet and headed out the door, slamming it on the way out.

Narcotic addicts seek their fix any way they can get it: from other addicts, on the street-or from a doctor. They often invent stories of pain, which, from frequent practice, become elaborate and highly believable tales. Sometimes they score big, sometimes just a limited supply, or sometimes they strike out.

After a few times of being suckered into prescribing narcotics for addicts, physicians usually develop a "gut" feeling about who those people are: patients with pain that's impossible to pinpoint, pain that doesn't respond to the non-narcotic treatments, patients who request a "drug of choice." Of course, the patient, if confronted with the physician's suspicions, will vehemently deny them and rain curses down upon her. Naturally, the physician resents being manipulated into abetting what is basically an illegal activity and which could jeopardize her license to practice medicine.

- *Do* expect your physician to be reluctant to prescribe narcotics if you're a new patient.

- *Don't* expect your physician to give you large amounts of refillable prescriptions of narcotics for pain.

- *Do* see your physician regularly for check-ups if you have a condition requiring periodic use of narcotics.

- *Do* realize that pharmacies keep close track of prescriptions for narcotics, and may notify your doctor if your usage seems excessive-or the police if the prescription appears to be forged.

The Doctor Shopper

Celia Conway looked distraught as Dr. Jodi Fleisch entered the room. "Oh, thank heavens!" the silver-haired Celia exclaimed as she looked the young physician up and down. "I hope I've finally found a doctor who can help me. They told me you just got out of training, so I'm hoping you've still got the brains to figure me out," she said, then laughed nervously.

"I'll certainly try," the physician said, also rather nervously. She was confident in her own intelligence and skills, but this patient was already sounding like a bit of a challenge. "Why don't you tell me about your problem?"

"I'll give you the condensed version; I don't think you've got time for the whole story. I've been having this pain in my left side ever since Christmas, and my regular doctor, Dr. Jamison Clark, didn't have the least idea what was causing it. Well, poor dear, he's older than I am and he's probably half-senile, if you want to know the truth. So then I saw his partner, Dr. Meeks, who took a bunch of tests and still couldn't find out what the problem was. And then I went to a doctor my sister recommended, another old man who just wanted to do a lot more tests, so I thought I'd come to see you and find out if you can get to the bottom of this."

"*Probably not*," thought Dr. Fleisch, discouraged by the odds, but said, "I'll do my best."

After taking a thorough history and doing a physical exam, she managed to convince Celia of the need to get the records of the treatment she'd already received, and to make a follow-up visit. But when, on the follow-up, Dr. Fleisch admitted she still wasn't sure what the problem was, Celia announced as she left the office, "Well, you've had your chance. I guess I'll just have to go down the list of doctors in the phone book one by one until I find someone who knows what they're doing."

At that moment Dr. Fleisch wished her last name had been Zeligman.

We've all heard stories–true stories–of patients who've visited doctor after doctor until they "finally found someone who found out what the real problem was." Often that's because the patient has a very unusual condition that is difficult to diagnose. Often, however, it's simply because the patient did not follow up with the initial physician.

For example, I've seen a number of patients treated for rashes that were initially thought to be caused by a fungus, but which on further evaluation were found to be caused by something else, like eczema. Then, when the patients get better with the new and appropriate treatment, they think I'm brilliant and the previous doctor(s) stupid. In reality, I used the knowledge of the failure of the previous diagnosis and treatment to go an obvious further step in the evaluation, one which the original doctor would have taken had the patient only returned to her. This is an example of why continuity of care is important. Shopping around may be the best way to get a great dress, but it's not the best way to get a good diagnosis.

- *Do* realize that not every medical problem can be solved in one visit, no matter how good your doctor is.

- *Do* follow up with your doctor as directed.

- *Do* ask your doctor about getting a second opinion if several visits have not been helpful, and do expect your doctor to be open to helping you see another physician.

- *Do* bring records of your previous tests and treatments if you see another doctor about your problem.

The New Guru

Joanie Ewing looked very serene as Dr. Marge Kahn walked into the exam room. The young sheet music store worker was sitting with the back of her hands laid on her thighs, and her eyes closed. It was hard for Dr. Kahn to imagine that Joanie was here for the problem the nurse had written in the chart: "severe headaches."

"Joanie," said the doctor, "I'm sorry to interrupt your meditation, but I'd like to talk to you about your headaches." She went through her standard list of questions, receiving mostly negative responses, until she got to the one about "recent stresses."

Joanie drew a deep breath. "My husband left me in November for a man, and I lost my job last month, but I'm at total inner peace now–really. I've been following the teaching of Pranawatan. I'm not only getting in touch with my inner life, but my past lives as well. What I'm experiencing lately is a sharp pain encircling my neck that feels like it's going to cut my head off. I think maybe the headaches are because I found out recently that I was beheaded during the French Revolution."

"Oh, were you Marie Antoinette?"

"No," said Joanie, missing the sarcasm entirely. "I think I was one of the lower nobility, but I did have a lovely chateau right outside of Paris."

Just as Dr. Kahn felt ready to burst out laughing, Joanie leaned forward and adopted a deadly serious tone. "You should become a follower of Pranawatan, too." Reaching into her handbag, she withdrew a gold-colored pamphlet entitled: "The Teachings of Pranawatan: Making Your Many Lives One," and handed it to Dr. Kahn. "If you follow him, he can help you as much as he's helped me."

"*In that case,*" thought Dr. Kahn, "*I'd better burn this.*"

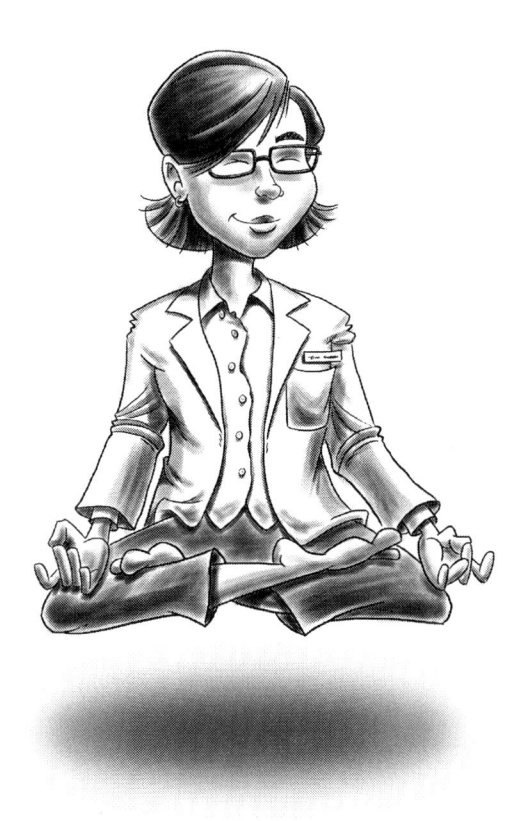

Spirituality is a necessity to the health of human beings. The physical, intellectual, emotional, and spiritual aspects of our lives must each be nurtured in order for the whole organism to function properly. Prayer has been found in a number of medical studies to have a powerful, positive effect on healing, not only when the patient herself prays, but even when others pray *for* the patient, in the absence of the patient's knowledge. On the other hand, there are times when specific religious practices may conflict with medical advice, as with Muslims who fast and can't take daytime medications during the month of Ramadan, or Jehovah's Witnesses who can't receive blood.

So in evaluating a person for depression, for instance, a psychiatrist will inquire into the religious background of the patient and also ask about any belief system and spiritual resources the patient has. If the patient has a belief system but is not connected with a particular church or other group, the physician may properly suggest that the patient seek out or join such a group. It would not be appropriate, however, for the doctor to use this opportunity to try to "convert" a vulnerable nonbeliever or coerce her into becoming a member of her own church. Likewise, a patient should not use the intimacy of the physician-patient encounter to proselytize the doctor. It's her duty to save your health, but not yours to save her soul.

- *Do* share your belief system and religious values with your physician if she asks.
- *Don't* expect the physician to share the same beliefs as you.
- *Do* expect the physician not to be dismissive or judgmental about your beliefs, but rather to support you in strengthening those beliefs if they will help you.

Ponce De Leon

With her broad-brimmed Mexican straw hat and neon-blue sunglasses, Claire Sanderson looked like she was ready for a day at the beach rather than a day at the doctor's office. As Dr. Lydia Bentley entered the room, Claire doffed the hat but not the sunglasses, which had prescription lenses. "Hello!" said Claire. "Ever since you sent me to that dermatologist, I've been avoiding the sun like poison. I feel like I'm turning into a vampire. But she told me I've got several pre-cancerous lesions on my face, and I'm not about to let things get worse. So here it is only April, and I'm already covered with sunscreen."

"Try not to get too paranoid," Dr. Bentley advised. "Certainly it's a good idea to avoid further sun damage, but most of the skin problems you have now are from years and years of sun exposure–and from the effects of aging, too, of course."

"I'm not *that* old, doctor," Claire said, frowning.

"Sorry, but I'm no kid myself–I'm six years older than you are." But the doctor didn't say that even at 51 she *looked* younger than her patient, who had been a lifeguard as a college student and a sun worshiper all her life, until now.

"I wanted to ask you about melatonin," said Claire. "Do you think it can keep people young?"

"I've never seen any convincing data that it helps slow down aging. But if you want to try it, go ahead."

"That doesn't sound very encouraging. Isn't there anything else I can try? What about sheep placenta cream?" she said with a laugh.

But Dr. Bentley gave a sober response. "There aren't any miracle drugs that I know of."

"Sometimes I think you doctors know the secret of eternal youth and you're just keeping it from the rest of us so you don't go out of business."

"If that were true," said Dr. Bentley, tugging at a lock of her gray-streaked hair, "this would still be brown."

Ponce de Leon was neither the first nor the last seeker of the fountain of youth. Judging from the billions of dollars spent each year on such things as plastic surgery, hair coloring, vitamins, melatonin, and other products, many of us still believe in that elusive dream.

Aging is a process that is intrinsic to every living organism. Nothing is alive now that will be alive forever (at least in *this* world). Whether we take the position that this is the design of God or of evolution, it's a simple fact, and it remains, even if you don't like it. Physicians don't like getting older any better you do, and sometimes we follow the same unsubstantiated, "crazy" youth-seeking regimens our patients do.

If there ever is a cure for old age, we physicians will be first in line, but we *will* share the news.

- *Do* follow a healthy lifestyle.
- *Do* avoid excessive sun exposure and smoking, which lead to premature wrinkling and aging of the skin. You may not be able to slow down aging, but you can speed it up.
- *Do* take anti-oxidant vitamins if you like, but realize that their effects on forestalling aging are not yet proven.
- *Do* see a plastic surgeon or dermatologist if you'd like; she can reverse some of the *effects* of aging.
- *Do* expect your doctor to help keep you healthy, but *don't* expect her to keep you young.

Remember, good health means you're dying at the normal rate.

The Doctor Idolizer

After living in Cincinnati for most of her 55 years, there were many things that Jeanine Patterson hated to leave behind when she and her husband Phil moved to Cleveland. His corporation was downsizing and closing the outlying offices, and Phil, still a few years from retirement, was lucky to get an offer to go to headquarters. Still, they were leaving their beautiful home with its new kitchen, the yard and garden with plants that had finally matured into full splendor–and her doctor. Dr. Abraham Morse had delivered her three children, had seen her family through numerous hospitalizations and countless office visits, and had even persuaded Phil to quit smoking.

After moving into their new house, Jeanine had developed a persistent cough that she blamed on all the dust that had been kicked up moving furniture and boxes. But four weeks later, after daily vacuuming, she was still coughing. Phil had been nagging her to see a doctor, but she couldn't imagine seeing someone other than Dr. Morse. She was happy with her new hairdresser, baker, and florist, but finding a new physician somehow smacked of betrayal, like going out looking for a new husband. The thought of hopping on a plane to pay Dr. Morse a visit seemed only slightly ridiculous to her. She'd put off calling him because she dreaded the advice she expected to hear: "Find a new doctor, dear." But one day after her cough had kept her (and Phil) up half the night, she found herself on the phone, trying to extort a diagnosis and treatment from Dr. Morse.

"I really think you should go see someone there in Cleveland," said the doctor. "I can't listen to your lungs over the telephone."

"But nobody here could be as good as you."

"Now, I, uh, doubt that," he stammered.

"And nobody knows me like you do. Last time I had that awful bronchitis, the antibiotic you prescribed worked like a charm. If you'd just call me in a prescription, I'm sure I'd be better in no time."

"Well, I don't know…"

"Oh, please, please. But you know I'll do whatever you say."

"Alright, but only if you promise to see someone if you're not better in 48 hours."

"It's a deal. Dr. Morse, you're the best!"

But she wasn't so sure about that when, two days later, she was laying in a bed in the hospital, with a diagnosis of congestive heart failure, not a respiratory infection.

Physicians enjoy admiration and praise as much as anyone else, and certainly it's appropriate to voice your heartfelt thanks to your doctor if you feel he's doing a good job. Physicians know they aren't God, even though people often accuse them of thinking they are. But the truth is, many people would like them to be gods–all-powerful beings who can cure diseases with a wave of their magic wands, if only their supplicants are faithful and ardent in their devotion. Doctor idolizers tend to revere men more frequently than women–female physicians being seen as nurturing, mother figures, and males as god-like power figures with thunderbolts in their hands. The worshipers throw themselves at the feet of these gods, cling to them, and follow them unquestioningly wherever they go. But blind devotion can lead you down the wrong path, so keep your eyes open and be ready to part ways when it's time to do so.

- *Do* have a primary care doctor who can coordinate or keep track of all your health care needs, but *don't* expect your doctor to be able to take care of all your needs all of the time by himself.

- *Do* realize that while your relationship with your physician is special, other doctors are available to help you when you need it.

- *Do* try to see the same doctor as much as possible to improve the continuity of your care.

- *Do* see a different doctor if your regular doctor is not available to see you within a reasonable period of time.

"Please Excuse Johnny From School Today"

Johnny Mennick looked like the picture of health: a muscular young man with a broad grin and a glowing acne-free complexion. At a glance, Dr. Lucille Yantz certainly couldn't guess what he was doing in her office.

"Not feeling well today, Johnny?"

"Oh, I'm okay now, but Tuesday I was, like, death warmed over. My throat killed and I had this major pain in my sinuses. I felt so bad I, like, missed one of my final exams at Clermont College. I wanna reschedule it, but my professor needs a note from you that says I was sick."

"Why didn't you come in on Tuesday?"

"I was, uh, too sick to leave the house."

"Uh-huh. Well, all I can give you is a note stating you were in to see me today. The rest is between you and your professor."

"Are you saying I'm lying?"

"No. All I'm saying is that I can't verify an illness that I never saw. Look, I could write something to the effect of 'patient reports having been ill on Tuesday.' Would that work for you?"

"Sure. Just put it on something that, like, looks official, so he doesn't think I faked it."

Sighing to herself as she obligingly handed him the note–with her office letterhead prominently displayed at the top–she felt more like his mother than his doctor.

Medical excuses for school and work can put your physician in an awkward position between you and your teacher or employer. Of course, your doctor's first duty is to you–even if she happens to work for the same school or employer–but that doesn't mean she has any power to make them rearrange your exam schedule or your job duties. If you do request a statement from your physician, make sure you're clear about what information you want released–there may be some details you'll want to keep confidential.

- *Don't* expect the physician to verify details of an illness that's no longer present when you see her.
- *Do* try to come in *during* your illness, if you're going to need a statement for your instructor or employer.

- *Don't* expect your physician to get you out of an exam for which you haven't studied or a work duty you find unpleasant.

The Antibiotic Addict

"I've got a terrible cold," said Mr. Jerald James, a 43-year-old self-employed roofer, "but if you give me some antibiotics, it'll fix me right up. I just can't afford to be laid up sick right now; it's almost spring and I'll be workin' 70 hours a week pretty soon." He wiped his raw, red nose with a damp handkerchief, and then sneezed as his physician tried to dodge his spray–she didn't want to be sick either.

Dr. Sharon Dernier's exam showed that his nasal lining was beefy red and swollen, with copious clear secretions, and his cervical lymph nodes were slightly enlarged. But otherwise the findings were unremarkable. "Looks like you've got a viral upper respiratory infection," she told him.

"That sounds pretty bad," said the patient. "What are you gonna give me? Last time I got penicillin it didn't seem to work too good. I think I need something stronger."

"*Oh-oh. Here we go again*," she thought. "The trouble is, Mr. James, antibiotics don't work for viral infections. They're only effective for bacterial infections like strep throat."

"So you're tellin' me there's nothin' I can do for this?"

"Well, no. There certainly are things that you can do to help with the symptoms–a decongestant for your runny nose, for instance."

"Then why did my old doctor prescribe antibiotics for me every time I got a cold?"

"Good question."

"Please, doctor," he begged, but with hostility rising through his plea, "you've got to give me some antibiotics!"

Suddenly she felt like she was dealing with a heroin addict–and denying him his fix.

The "common cold" is defined as a viral upper respiratory tract infection. The simple fact is that no antibiotic is effective for a virus–that's NO antibiotic, period. Most colds last about a week, so if your doctor prescribes 7 to 10 days worth of antibiotics and you have a viral cold, it's going to get better—not because of the medicine, but simply because the illness has run its course. The body's own immune system has eliminated the infection.

So it would seem a simple matter that doctors should stop prescribing antibiotics for colds. But SOME respiratory infections are bacterial and indeed can be treated effectively with antibiotics: many pneumonias, sinus infections, ear infections, and of course streptococcal pharyngitis ("strep throat"). So how does the physician decide whether the infection is viral or bacterial? Minimal fever, clear secretions and multiple symptoms (nasal congestion, sore throat, cough, achy feeling) are typical for viruses; high fever, dark discolored secretions, and localized symptoms (such as pressure over the left cheek from a sinus infection) are often encountered in bacterial infections. But these are generalizations, and these sets of symptoms and findings often overlap. Even lab tests like blood counts and throat cultures are not completely reliable.

But an antibiotic can't hurt, right? Wrong. People still die every year from severe reactions to antibiotics, and many people have side effects like diarrhea or yeast infections. There's also a growing concern that over-prescription of antibiotics is helping to contribute to the development of "superbugs," bacteria that have become resistant to most antibiotics. The saying "that which doesn't kill us only makes us stronger," can be applied to bacteria as well as humans.

So why do physicians often prescribe antibiotics for "colds"? Since we can't be absolutely certain that a particular cold is viral, one motivation to prescribe antibiotics is "just in case" the infection if bacterial. But far more common is the irresistible pressure from our patients to prescribe them. After the discovery of penicillin, which became the miracle drug to treat infections, the myth developed that antibiotics could cure anything infectious. Myth is often more powerful–and hope-inspiring–than fact; we all want to believe there's a cure when we're feeling miserable. We doctors also want to believe we have something that can help you, and on top of that, respiratory infections are the single most common reason for a visit to a primary care doctor's office. If everyone with a cold stopped coming to see their doctors, our business would drop off. But that doesn't mean we should just give you what you want so you'll keep coming back.

So if your doctor says you probably have a virus and that antibiotics won't help, it's not that she wants you to suffer or feels like you're wasting her time–she just doesn't want to expose you to the unnecessary side effects and expense of antibiotics.

- *Don't* presume that every time you go in to the office for a respiratory infection that you will receive a prescription for an antibiotic.
- *Do* realize that antibiotics are not entirely innocuous substances. They can cause side effects and allergic reactions.

- *Do* contact your physician or return to the office if your symptoms change, which means the treatment may also need to be changed.

MISCELLANEOUS MISUNDERSTANDINGS

The Waiting Room Magazine Bandit

Shirley Claghorn hadn't noticed the fact that it was 20 minutes past her appointment time and the doctor still wasn't ready for her. After solving the newspaper's crossword puzzle, she became absorbed in the waiting room copy of *Architectural Digest*, trying to figure out how she could remodel her kitchen to resemble the one belonging to the Hollywood celebrity featured in the magazine–but at a fraction of the cost. When the nurse finally called her name, she was almost annoyed to have to interrupt her reading. While no one was looking, it was easy to slip the magazine into her oversized Mexican leather handbag; she could finish the article later at her leisure.

Dr. Yong Cha Soo greeted her patient, and then spied the top of the magazine sticking out of Shirley's bag. Pointing, the doctor said, "That's a great issue. I especially like the old mansion on Martha's Vineyard. Maybe someday my house will look like that–after the kids leave."

Shirley smiled and said, "I, uh, was planning to put it back before I left."

"I'm sure you were." Then wrinkling her brow, Dr. Soo said, "I've just never been able to figure out how we can start the week with twenty magazines and have only ten by Friday."

Shirley had no answer to the doctor's puzzle.

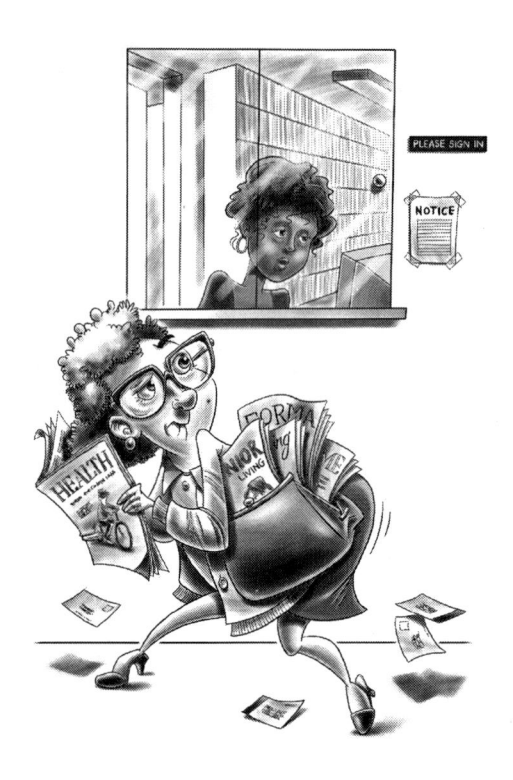

So what's the big deal? It's just an old magazine that one of the employees brought in, probably six months to a year out-of-date. But it's still property belonging to the office. You don't take the tongue blades and otoscopes home with you, do you? Let's hope not. Often, someone had to buy those magazines. But sometimes, free or "complimentary" copies of certain publications are sent to physicians expressly for their waiting rooms. Still, even those free reading materials are for *everybody* to share. Have you ever been in a waiting room where the only magazines left were a two-year-old copy of *Sports Illustrated* and a torn-up *Reader's Digest*? All the others had "walked off"–and then the wait for the doctor seemed even longer than usual.

- *Do* leave the magazines for everyone to read.

- *Do* copy down any information you'd like to keep, either by jotting it down or having a copy made. All physician offices have copiers, and usually the staff will be glad to make you a copy at a minimal charge.

- *Do* ask if you can borrow the magazine, and then *do* bring it back.

- *Do* ask if you can keep the magazine, if it's old and they might be getting ready to pitch it anyway, but be prepared to hear "no."

- *Do* bring in magazines of your own from time to time to share with the office.

"I'm Allergic To Something"

Jessie Day, a 20-year-old college junior majoring in journalism, had a term paper due in two days and had been staying up late to finish it–and drinking coffee to stay awake. So when she began feeling like she had to urinate every hour, she wasn't surprised, and simply attributed it to the caffeine. But later, when her urine also began to burn, she knew she had a bladder infection, an all-too-common occurrence for her. Sometimes she would call her doctor and the doctor would just phone in a prescription to her pharmacy, but having just transferred from another school, she came in for the first time to her new school's student health clinic.

After listening to Jessie's symptoms, Dr. Marisa Romana was reviewing her past medical history. "I'll be putting you on some antibiotics if the urine test confirms an infection.

Are you allergic to anything that you know of?"

"No. I mean yes, but I'm not sure what the name of it is."

"Well, do you at least know what *type* of medicine it was–an antibiotic or a pain pill or a stomach medicine or what?"

"No, I just can't remember."

"Okay, then do you remember what happened–did you break out in a rash or have trouble breathing or stomach upset?"

"I think I got a rash. What's the big deal?"

"It's important because if you were truly allergic to that medicine, and I prescribed it for you, you could have a serious, even fatal, allergic reaction. We could try to call your physician at the other student health center."

"It was shut down this year because of the budget crunch."

"Then how about your family physician?"

"He's dead. I don't know who has the records."

"Well then, we'll need you to take the medicine while you're here and keep an eye on you for 20 minutes to make sure that you don't have a bad reaction–or if you do, we can resuscitate you."

Growing visibly pale, Jessie said, "Guess I should have learned what I was allergic to."

Allergic reactions can run the gamut, from the annoying sniffles some people get from spring pollens in the air, to the life-threatening anaphylactic shock that can occur after a bee sting. Allergies involve an interaction between the allergic substance and IgE antibodies, which can trigger a cascade of other molecular reactions resulting in hives, asthma, and shock.

Other adverse effects of medications, termed side effects, are generally milder but occasionally can be severe: seizures, bone marrow suppression, cardiac arrhythmias. While your doctor will routinely keep track of any bad reactions you've had to medicines, it's important for you to know the name of the drug and the nature of your reaction, and to tell any doctor you see about it.

- *Do* know what medications you're allergic to.
- *Do* know the difference between an allergy and a side effect.
- *Do* carry an identification bracelet if you have a potentially deadly allergy.
- *Don't* expect your doctor to want to gamble with prescribing medications if you don't know what you're allergic to.

"It's A Little White Pill…"

Virginia McCafferty had to be doing something right. At the age of 93, she still had her wits about her, most of her teeth, and a healthy (and kind) heart. Her only formula for living a long life was to get up each day and do it all over again; she didn't pay attention to the details. So when she outlived her doctor and had to see a new one for a refill of her arthritis medicine, she expected the visit to go just like all her previous visits to ol' Dr. Johnson.

"The trouble is," said young Dr. Johnny Ciccione, "I can't refill your medicine if I don't know what it is."

"It's a little white pill," she said, confident that would settle it.

"Well, that narrows it down to a few hundred medicines. Look, we can call your pharmacy and find out what you're on, but you really ought to know the names of your medicines."

"I guess I could try, but I've got more important things to remember, like the name of my new great-great grandchild: Virginia!"

Medicines come in all shapes, sizes, colors, and forms—from capsules to tablets to liquids. White (with its implication of purity) is the most common, with pastels of pink and blue and yellow close behind. Green (with its connotation of poison) is a rare color, and black (with its funereal association) likewise is a rare shade for drugs (at least the legal kind).

- *Do* know the names of your medications and what they're for.

- *Do* carry a list of your medications and illnesses–in case you have trouble remembering them, or in case you're in an accident or rendered unconscious.

- *Don't* expect your physician to know your medication by simply describing its size and color.

The Handshaker

Jerry Case was a car salesman by trade; he knew his cars and he knew how to shake hands. Handshaking was an art form to him. He could caress a lonely widow's hand, give a neutral non-sexist shake to a businesswoman, and square off with a macho man as if in a prelude to an arm-wrestling match. The touch of the skin, with its variations of warmth and dampness, transmitted the information to him: "I'm a nervous first-time buyer," "I'm just window-shopping," or "I'm hot to buy."

But sometimes people were reluctant to shake his hand. This struck him not only as unfriendly, but downright un-American. So it was puzzling to Jerry when as he greeted his internist, Henry Thorsen, that the doctor seemed hesitant about extending his hand. Of course, Jerry had retracted his own hand just a moment ago–to cover a violent coughing fit.

Handshaking, a seemingly innocuous form of greeting, is a custom that is possibly responsible for spreading more colds and infections than any other behavior. The hands themselves aren't the problem, of course–it's what they come in contact with. When we have a cold we're constantly blowing our noses and coughing into our hands, and inoculating them with secretions that have infectious organisms in them. Then the hands go to doorknobs, eating utensils—and other hands!

Doctors should–and do–wash their hands between patients. But we're susceptible to infections just like you, and would like to avoid them, just like you. So, when you're in the office, turn your head and cover your mouth when you cough.

There are alternatives to the handshake. The "elbow bump" may look a little funny, but if it becomes culturally accepted, could prevent a lot of infections. The "fist bump" is cleaner than the handshake but could still pose a small risk. And of course a nice big smile and nod of the head is a friendly greeting that involves no contact—and no risk—at all.

- *Do* wash your hands if you're blowing your nose or coughing into your hand.
- *Don't* be offended if your physician nods or just says hello rather than shakes your hand.
- *Do* expect your doctor to wash up before and/or after your visit.

- *Don't* try to shake hands as you're leaving if your doctor has just washed up.

The Soap Opera

The Margolecz family, recent immigrants from the war-torn former country of Yugoslavia, was busy adjusting to their new home and new country. Learning the language was the most pressing priority. As usual, the children were picking it up much faster than their parents, so when Kordy Margolecz, a 53-year-old former electrician, came down with a high fever, 9-year-old Janus came in to the office as the interpreter.

Smiles greeted Dr. Jim Kinshaw as he entered the room–but so did a powerful stench. The triangular interview, from doctor to son to father and back again, took longer than usual, and by the time it was over, Dr. Kinshaw could barely stand to be in the room any longer. Kordy's custom in his home country, where his house had no hot running water, was to bathe only once per week, and though the family was now in an apartment with hot water available at the turn of a tap, he saw no reason to change his custom.

Dr. Kinshaw had been seeing a lot of influenza cases lately, and after a brief exam of the patient's ears, throat, and chest, concluded he had the flu. "If he doesn't get better in the next couple of days," the doctor advised Janus, "bring your father back, but have him take a bath first."

Although puzzled by the instructions to bathe–thinking it might be some kind of medical treatment–Kordy dutifully bathed prior to reappearing two days later when his fever persisted. This time, after a more complete (and more pleasant) exam, the diagnosis was obvious: a secondary bacterial infection of a severe case of tinea pedis ("athlete's foot"). A combination of oral antibiotics and topical antifungals quickly cleared up a problem that was initially overlooked due to the "olfactory factor."

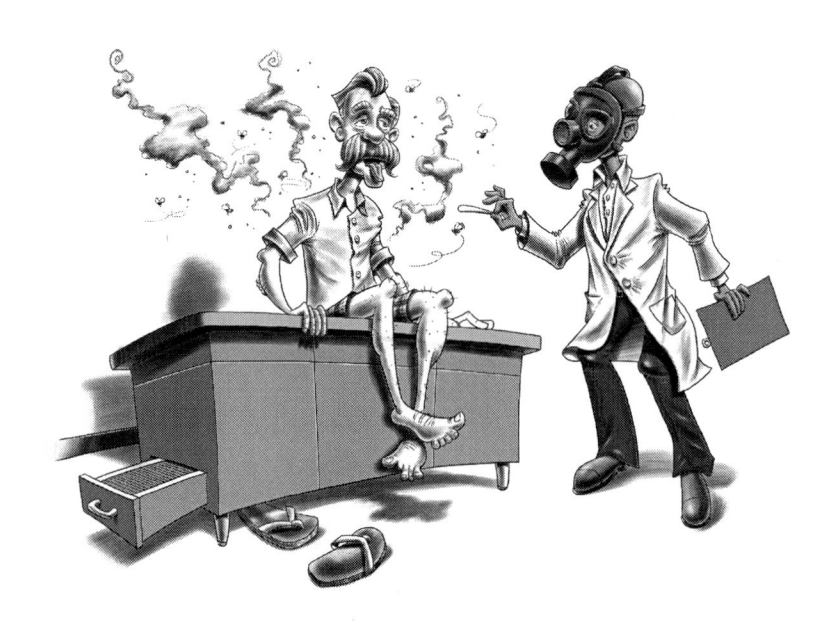

Daily bathing and the use of deodorants is part of American culture–at least since the late 20th century. A hundred years ago, before indoor plumbing became commonplace, bathing was a major chore. If you had to pump the water, haul it inside, heat it on a stove, and then dump it out again, how often would you bathe?

Some people even thought of bathing as unhealthful, washing away the body's natural protective layer. Indeed, too much bathing and hand washing can lead to dry skin. Regular hand washing helps to reduce the risk of acquiring and spreading colds, hepatitis, and other infections. But mainly, when we speak of bathing, we're referring to a social custom. And American noses are now accustomed to being greeted by the smells of soap and perfume, not sweat and body odor.

- *Do* shower or bathe on the day of your visit, or at least wash the part of your body likely to be examined.
- *Don't* expect extra cologne or perfume to take the place of a bath–in fact, it may create an additional offense to the nose.

The Fashion Model

Denise Hathaway loved to wear tight jeans–after all, she looked great in them. So the young woman wore them everywhere–to class, on dates, shopping–and to the doctor's office. Today she had come to see her pediatrician, Dr. Mark Lopez. Even though she was almost 20, she hated the thought of having to see a strange new doctor, and Dr. Lopez rewarded her by continuing to see her; though she wasn't a baby, she wasn't old yet, either.

For the past two weeks she'd been noticing a few spots on her legs. "Let me take a look at them," said the physician.

"No problem," said Denise, but there was a problem. She tugged mightily at her jeans but couldn't get them rolled up past her calves. "There's a couple of them," she said, pointing to a pair of small reddish lesions.

"Doesn't look like anything specific."

"There are a couple more up higher, but I can't get my jeans up that high."

It was a busy day in the office, and Dr. Lopez didn't want to have to wait for her to disrobe and put on an exam gown. "It's probably an irritation from shaving. Try this cortisone cream, and let me know if it doesn't get better," he said as he wrote out a prescription.

One week later, Denise was back. "It's no better," she said. "Maybe worse." Being on her way to a job interview this time, she had abandoned her usual attire for a navy blue dress.

This time, Dr. Lopez could see a lesion on Denise's right knee which was larger than the ones lower down, and which resembled a scaly ring. Now the diagnosis was obvious–ringworm. "It's a fungal infection," he explained as he handed her a new prescription–for an antifungal cream.

While it's not necessary to be totally naked for every examination by a doctor, adequate exposure is certainly important. The physician will generally want to see not just the specific part of your body that's bothering you, but the adjacent regions as well, in case there are clues to your diagnosis or complications visible elsewhere. If you have a sore throat and head congestion, your doctor will look not only in your throat and ears, but listen to your lungs as well, to check for pneumonia–they're all part of the respiratory tract. So wear a blouse you can lift up rather than a one-piece dress. If you've injured your knee, wear some exercise shorts under your pants, so you can quickly doff the pants and expose the area above and below the knee. And if you're having eye trouble, be prepared to remove your contact lenses; bring your case and solutions.

- *Do* wear clothing that is easily removed or that exposes the part of your body which needs to be examined.

- *Do* disrobe and put on an exam gown if requested to do so by the nurse; the less time spent waiting for you to disrobe, the more time your physician has to examine you.

- *Do* keep on your undergarments if you feel uncomfortable not having them on.

- *Do* put your coat on or ask for a blanket if you feel cold.

"My Chiropractor Says…"

"My chiropractor says my neck is crooked and I need to have it adjusted periodically," said Len Pearson, a 37-year-old truck driver, holding his neck with both hands, as if to keep it from falling off his shoulders. "The adjustments help a lot, but I think my neck went out this morning as I was unloading the truck. My chiropractor's on vacation in Jamaica right now, so I wondered if you could crack it for me."

"Well, Mr. Pearson, that's really not my specialty," replied his internist, Dr. Julia Dominguez. "But let me take a look and see what I can do for you."

"I suppose you'll just want to push a few pills at me," he pouted.

"Sometimes medication *can* be very helpful," she countered.

"No, thanks. I can show you right where he puts his fingers when he adjusts me…"

"Sorry, there are some things I just don't do."

"Huh," he grunted, straightening up a little so he could look her in the eye. "And I thought you doctors could do *anything*."

Chiropractic medicine and allopathic medicine both care for ailments, are practiced by health professionals, and require specialized training and licensing. Both have treated millions of patients over the years, patients who have benefited from their treatments and who swear by the talents of their care providers.

Allopathic medicine is finding that it needs to be open about other forms of care, not only chiropractic medicine, but acupuncture, herbal medicine, massage therapy, and others–keeping as a priority that which benefits the patients and not just the profession.

- *Do* expect that your physician will perform her own history and physical and form her own diagnosis, just like she would do if you were coming from another physician instead of your chiropractor.

- *Do* expect that your physician might want to repeat your X-rays; she may feel that different or additional views are needed.

- *Do* expect your physician to listen to your story of your chiropractic treatment and the results you experienced.

- *Don't* expect your chiropractor and your physician to necessarily advise the same kinds of treatments.

The Sensitive Stomach

Jenny Mars, a 17-year-old cheerleader for the Kinnesaw High School Rams, had fallen off the top of the pyramid during a recent practice and considered herself lucky to have walked away with only a sprained wrist. But it was her left hand, and since that was her dominant hand, it was painful just to write or do many of her daily activities. She showed up in her pediatrician's office requesting some relief.

"Ibuprofen should be helpful for both the pain and the inflammation," said her physician, Dr. Linda Goren.

"That stuff just tears my stomach up, doctor. I have a sensitive stomach."

Dr. Goren glanced back at Jenny's chart and saw that under the section labeled "Allergies and Side Effects" no less than five medications were listed: penicillin, erythromycin, tetracycline, codeine, and prochlorperazine. Except for penicillin–which had given her hives–all the medications had "stomach upset" listed as the adverse reaction she had experienced. Ironically, the prochlorperazine had even been prescribed to try to *relieve* her stomach upset. "In that case, it looks like we'd better stick with acetaminophen," concluded Dr. Goren.

"I've already tried that," said Jenny, "and it's not helping."

So Dr. Goren prescribed a pain reliever with codeine. Sure enough, Jenny called to the office the next day complaining, "That medicine is making me terribly nauseated, doctor. I'd rather just live with the pain and see if my wrist won't get better on its own."

"Fine," replied Dr. Goren. "Come see me again if you're not better in another week." Sighing, she opened Jenny's chart to the section on "Allergies and Side Effects" and added another one to the list.

Some people claim to have a "sensitive stomach," while others say they have an "iron stomach." Certainly different individuals can have very different reactions to the same medications; one person can take erythromycin, for example, with no noticeable reaction, while another may become violently ill. There are some who seem to experience gastrointestinal side effects to nearly everything they ingest–these are the ones with the "sensitive stomachs." This can be problematic in treating a patient because it can result in a long list of medications to be avoided, and elimination of many treatment options.

"Stomach upset" symptoms like nausea or loose stools, without hives or wheezing, are not usually due to an allergy, but can be a side effect of nearly any oral medication. (People even get stomach upset with placebo pills.) Rarely these side effects can be severe–even life-threatening, such as *Clostridium difficile* diarrhea from antibiotics–but usually they are mild and don't necessarily warrant discontinuing the medication.

- *Do* expect that minor gastrointestinal side effects may occur with many medications.

- *Do* contact your physician if the side effects are troublesome.

- *Do* discontinue your medication if symptoms are severe (such as repeated vomiting, severe diarrhea, abdominal cramping) and contact your physician.

Ring-A-Ding-Ding

As he stepped into the exam room, Dr. Gregory Lee could see that his next patient, Crystal Fairchild, loved hardware. She had on a silver necklace, large red hoop earrings, a laptop computer balanced on her knees, and a cell phone attached to her right ear. All of this contrasted with the lightness of her features: her soft, blond hair, her pale blue eyes, and her sweet voice, which Dr. Lee could hear greeting not himself, but a friend of hers on the phone line.

"Hi, Danielle!" Laughing, she continued, "Say, I know I just got hold of you, but I'm in the doctor's office and he just walked in, and I really have to go. Uh-huh. Oh, my gosh, you are so kidding! I can't believe it. But that is so like Carter. I don't know anybody else who would even think of doing that. Yeah, well, I want all the details later, but like I said, I really gotta go. Well, sure, I'll be there tonight. I'm just here for my check-up—don't worry, you're not going to catch anything. Oh, but I talked to Sandra earlier and she can't make it . Yeah. Uh-huh." Noticing Dr. Lee out of the corner of her eye, Crystal said, "I'll call you in a little while. No. I'm hanging up. Bye." Brightly, without any real tone of apology, she said, "I'm sorry about that, Dr. Lee."

"No problem," replied Dr. Lee, even though that's not what he was thinking. "Now, let's see. You're here for your regular gynecological checkup. How are you feeling? Anything you need to discuss with me today?"

Crystal was about to answer when the sounds of a hip-hop song started to emanate from the phone. "Oops, that's mine." Without waiting for Dr. Lee to comment, she flipped open the phone and said, "Teresa? Yeah, I know it's you—I've got you on my caller ID. Listen, I'm in the doctor's office right now. No, not the waiting room, I'm in the office, and the doctor is standing right here. Yes, I know, Danielle just told me. No, she's not here with me. I just talked to her on the phone. Oh, my gosh, she didn't tell me that!"

While Crystal was busy talking, Dr. Lee opened the door gently and slid into the hall. "I'll be back in a few minutes, when you're available," he called over his shoulder.

Crystal, listening instead of talking on the phone at the moment, opened her mouth as if to say something, but the door was already shut before she could get it out.

Cell phones are everywhere in our society: at home, at work, in schools, in stores—and in doctors' offices. While cell phone use in your doctor's office may not be dangerous, like it is while driving, it can still impact the care you receive. Receiving or initiating calls while in the waiting room may be acceptable if you use a low voice (and don't mind having others overhear your conversation), but texting would be a better option. In the presence of your physician, pretend you're in a theater and turn off all electronic devices. It's not only rude to talk on your phone during your visit, but can waste the precious time allotted for you to communicate with your health care provider. Of course, it's fine for you to carry your cell phone with you. Sometimes it can even be very helpful for your visit—the doctor may need you to call a relative to check on your vaccination history or inquire about diseases that run in the family, or to have someone come pick you up because you're not feeling well.

- *Do* turn off your cell phone when in the office, especially when in the exam room.
- *Do* use text messaging if possible, if you must make a call, so that others are not disturbed by your conversation (or overhearing it).

"You Want To Do What?!"

In his 66 years, Charles Walters had been through a lot in the hands of doctors. He had his tonsils out at the age of 9, a broken arm set (without anesthesia!) at 17, a North Korean bullet removed from his lumbar spine at 20, a malignant mole taken off his neck at 45, and—just a year ago—both knees replaced by artificial joints. But never until now had he been asked to undergo something he dreaded even more: a rectal exam.

Dr. Benjamin Purdy, his new physician, was evaluating his complaint of having to get up four times every night to urinate. "Your urine looks clear under the microscope," said Dr. Purdy. "No sign of infection or diabetes. I suspect your prostate is enlarged, and so I need to do a rectal exam to check it out."

"You want to do what?!" asked the incredulous patient.

"A rectal exam. Surely you've had one done before, when you've had your yearly check-ups."

"Ah, I think check-ups are a waste of money. I only go to a doctor when something's wrong. And now I'm starting to wish I hadn't come in for this either."

"A rectal exam is really no big deal. I just insert a gloved, lubricated finger into the rectum, so I can feel for nodules or other abnormalities. It might cause a little cramping, kind of like a bowel movement in reverse."

"Well," said Charles, swallowing hard, "grease me up good, doc!"

As Charles bent forward over the exam table, Dr. Purdy moved in from behind to find Charles' buttocks squeezed together tightly. "Relax," he told the patient.

"Easy for you to say," replied Charles. He did manage to take a deep breath and release his tension enough to allow the exam to proceed. But when Dr. Purdy slid his forefinger into the patient's rectum, Mr. Walters yelped. "Owww! Take it out—it hurts!"

"It'll just take a sec..."

"Take it out now!" said Mr. Walters as he reached around and grabbed the physician's hand.

"Okay," said Dr. Purdy, as he pulled off his gloves. "I'll send you to the urologist. Let's just hope his fingers aren't any bigger than mine."

People have different levels of comfort with examination of different parts of their bodies. Nobody objects to a doctor looking in their ears; and most people say "aaah" readily when their throats are being examined (though it makes some people gag). But when it comes to the rectal exam, many people react negatively–and vociferously. Some anticipate it will be painful, and it's the tension from that fear which causes most of the pain. A doctor's finger is smaller than a typical bowel movement, and much better lubricated. For some people there also exists a sexual association with the act of penetration, and some men in particular seem to find the act "humiliating." These fears and feelings lead people to avoid mentioning rectal problems or to declining the rectal exam as part of a complete physical, thus potentially overlooking a significant medical problem.

- *Do* realize that rectal exams are a normal part of the evaluation of gastrointestinal, urinary, and pelvic problems.

- *Do* ask to have a nurse or assistant present during the exam, if that would make you more comfortable.

- *Do* have a rectal exam as part of your complete physical if recommended by your physician, as a screen for rectal cancer and other problems.

The Animal Lover

Kate Corning had been a cat owner since the age of 8–and an asthma patient since the age of 9. By the time she was taken to an allergist and found to be allergic to her cat, "Scooter" had already given birth to her first litter, and the Cornings had found one of the kittens too irresistible to give away. By the age of 15, Kate was taking an antihistamine and two different inhalers, but still having trouble breathing.

Her pediatrician, Dr. Sue Petrovsky, was getting a little frustrated. "You know, the next step in treatment would be oral steroids. They can interfere with your growth, make you gain weight, or give you ulcers. But you could avoid all that–maybe even get rid of all your medicines–if you'd give away your cats."

"No way," declared Kate. "They're my babies!"

"At least keep the cats out of your bedroom. Since you spend more time there than any other room of the house, that might be enough to make a difference."

"I've tried that, but they scratch at the door and meow until I let them in."

Dr. Petrovsky shrugged her shoulders. "I just hope *you* have nine lives, too."

Animals can be a source of fun and comfort–even a source of medical benefit. "Pet therapy" has been used in nursing homes, for instance, to calm patients and lower their blood pressure. Unfortunately, pets can also be a source of medical problems. Bites and scratches are an obvious danger, and pets can also carry disease-causing organisms that are transmissible to humans. They also shed dander, which can provoke allergic responses ranging from the merely annoying—sneezing and itchy eyes—to life-threatening asthma. Trouble is, by the time people realize they're allergic to their pets, they can't bear to part with them.

Your doctor can certainly prescribe medications to help counteract the allergies or other problems engendered by your pet, but she'll probably also advise you to reduce your exposure (by keeping the animal out of certain rooms, not spending as much time with it, or even giving it away), not because she hates pets, but because she wants you to get better.

- *Do* ask your doctor for a guide on how to "desensitize" your house by decreasing the amount of animal dander.

- *Do* keep your pets out of the bedroom if you're allergic to them. (Don't let them in even for a little while–the dander they leave behind lingers.)

- *Do* strongly consider not replacing an allergy-provoking pet when it dies.

- *Do* wash your hands before you prepare food if you've been handling your pet.

- *Don't* let infants and young children play around the litter box.

- *Don't* leave a young child unattended with a pet: either one could come to harm.

Patients Who Die

"Good afternoon, Mason!" said Dr. Harold Weinberger as he entered the room where a gaunt, elderly man hunched forward in his chair, laboring to breathe despite having an oxygen cannula in his nose. The cheery greeting was perhaps inappropriate, but it seemed to be all the doctor had to offer. The surgery hadn't gotten all the cancer, and the chemotherapy wasn't working either. Worst of all, thought the physician, he hadn't been able to get his patient to stop smoking, something that probably would have prevented this whole sad mess, if done years ago.

Mason Carr had been one of Dr. Weinberger's first patients when he started practice 40 years ago, and he continued to be one of the most loyal. The doctor had delivered Mason's children, and even two of his grandchildren, before giving up obstetrics. The physician had thought Mason was a goner 10 years ago when he had a major heart attack, but he pulled through and improved his heart health by exercising, losing weight, and giving up cholesterol-rich foods–but not cigarettes.

"What can I do for you today, Mason?" asked Dr. Weinberger, truly not knowing the answer.

"I want you to set me up with that hospice program you talked about earlier. I think I'm ready for it now."

"But there may be some additional treatments that Dr. Graber can recommend, or…"

"I don't want any more of his poisons."

"Maybe radiation therapy could…"

"Give it up, Harry. I have. I'm okay with dying. Listen—you've been a great doctor. Don't try to keep me alive just to prove you can do it."

Death is the Great Enemy of us all. Most people spend a lot of time worrying about it and trying to avoid it; a physician does the same and calls that his job.

There are many reasons physicians may be upset about a patient's death–besides the loss of a paying customer. The patient may have been someone the physician saw regularly enough to have developed a personal regard for him, and so will feel as if he's lost a friend. But even if it's someone he's never seen before–as with an accident victim who dies in the emergency room–physicians will hate to hand anyone over to the Grim Reaper. After all, the whole focus of their training is to keep people alive and well; anything less than that can make them feel like a failure. Some have objectified their professional roles to the extent that they feel the loss not worse than the loss of a chess game; others are devastated and find themselves questioning their own abilities. Death, when unexpected, is also considered a "bad result" and may provoke fear of a malpractice suit, even though the physician did nothing wrong. But death isn't always a bad thing; sometimes, as in the case of Mr. Carr, it can be a blessing.

- *Do* realize that in a patient's death, the physician may share (though to a lesser extent) your sense of loss.
- *Don't* automatically blame the doctor for a patient's death. He's not God and can only postpone death, not cure it.
- *Don't* die. (Good luck—we're all going for this one!)

Playtime In The Office

Peering through the aperture of Dr. Barry Green's ophthalmoscope, Tomas Mendez wondered what it was that doctors saw with these things. He held his hand in front of the instrument and turned a wheel which made different shapes and colors of light play across his palm.

"Good afternoon," said Dr. Green, striding into the room.

Tomas didn't seen to be the least bit embarrassed to be caught playing with the equipment, and nonchalantly replaced it in the recharging receptacle. He'd been having drainage from his left eye ever since flying back from his vacation in Costa Rica. Dr. Green took the ophthalmoscope and began to examine Tomas's eyes.

"What do you see?" asked the curious Tomas.

"Well, the light's a little weak from you having turned it on," he said, "but I'm looking at your fundus—the back of your eye—and it seems to be normal. The condition you have is just a superficial infection of the outer layer of your eye: conjunctivitis."

"I think it started after I got some sand in my eye and kept rubbing it."

"Uh-huh, that certainly could have done it. I'll put you on some eye drops which should help clear it up."

As he was writing the prescription, Tomas took the reflex hammer from the instrument table and began banging the front of his knees with it, eventually by chance hitting the patellar tendon in just the right spot to make his quadriceps contract and his knee extend.

"Hey, I got my knee jerk!" exclaimed Tomas, please to have discovered how the "toy" worked.

"So I see," said Dr. Green, handing him the prescription. "*'Jerk' is exactly the right word*," he thought.

As children we have a natural, selfish tendency to hoard our toys and to want no one else to play with them. And even though we are taught to share our dolls and video games, as we grow older and our toys change, we don't easily let someone else log onto our computer or drive our car or borrow the family dog.

A doctor's instruments may seem like toys–flashy little gadgets that can do fascinating things. But they're *not* toys, they're pieces of professional equipment which require certain skills to use properly. It's possible for you to break them, or inoculate them with your germs. And not only are they not toys, they're not *yours*, so kindly keep your "mitts" off them!

- *Don't* play with the office equipment.
- *Do* ask how something works if your curiosity is consuming you.
- *Do* realize that your hands have bacteria, viruses, and fungi on them that can be transmitted to the instruments and then to other patients.
- *Do* take a magazine or other pastime with you when the assistant seats you in the exam room, as you may still be waiting for the doctor for awhile; that way you'll be less tempted to play with the other things in the exam room.

Patients Who Don't Follow Up

"*So,*" thought Dr. Rita Barnhardt, as she glanced through the chart of her next patient, "*he finally made it back in.*" Mr. Cedric Hathaway, a 59-year-old retired plumber, was supposed to come in every month to get his blood pressure checked and his medication adjusted to the optimal level, but he hadn't been in for nearly half-a-year. "Hello, Mr. Hathaway," she greeted him. "Haven't seen you for quite awhile. I was starting to worry about you."

He leaned back and crossed his arms in front of him as if in self-defense. "I've been feeling fine. I may be retired, but I've got better things to do than to run to the doctor all the time to get my blood pressure checked."

"But I asked you to come just once a month. It's important to get your blood pressure under control even though you're not feeling ill. A stroke could be the first symptom you'd have!"

Mr. Hathaway was not rattled in the least. "Ah, you doctors are always tryin' to scare people. I wouldn't even be takin' this stuff if my wife didn't nag me about it every morning."

"Well," said Dr. Barnhardt, "if nagging works, I'll start, too."

Doctors want you to return to the office for follow-up visits on your health problems for a number of reasons. Sure, they want to maintain a busy schedule and keep the cash flow steady, but primarily, following up is an important part of your care.

For new conditions that are persisting, it's essential to do further evaluation and consider a different line of treatment. Even if you've gotten better, there may be important information–such as a mildly abnormal blood test drawn at your previous visit–which your physician needs to discuss with you. For chronic illnesses, it's necessary to continually fine-tune your treatment and to check for complications.

If you don't show up, the office staff or the physician himself may phone you to remind you of the need to reschedule. They're not hounding you–they're just trying to make sure you're doing well. That's their job!

- *Do* keep your follow-up appointments as scheduled.
- *Do* call to cancel and reschedule if you can't keep your follow-up appointment, and let the office personnel know how you're doing.

- *Do* ask the physician to explain if you're not sure why she's advising you to return to the office.

"Have I Got News For You!"

Rose Howe couldn't wait to see her doctor; she had big news for him. As soon as she entered the exam room, she began waving a piece of paper in the air. "Oh, Dr. Gladwyn, I'm so excited. I read this article today and I just had to bring it in and show you."

Dr. Dean Gladwyn took the paper from her and read the headline: "Peanut Oil Discovered to be Miracle Cure for Arthritis." Groaning inwardly, he asked, "What magazine did you get this from?"

"*The National Informer,*" Rose replied.

"Ah, not exactly *TheNew England Journal of Medicine,*" he said, trying to employ enough sarcasm to get his point across but without sounding angry.

"I don't believe all the stuff they write about aliens, but I think some of their stories must be reliable, otherwise how could they print them?"

"Good question," responded Dr. Gladwyn. "And I wish I knew the answer."

Reports of medical breakthroughs are daily fodder for the media, sometimes even claiming front-page status. A new anti-fat pill, a new cancer test, a new drug for arthritis, all seem to leap right from the laboratory into our living rooms, whether by television, newspaper, or magazine. Unfortunately, even in this brief transition, much of the information gets distorted or exaggerated or later is found to be unsubstantiated.

If your doctor isn't aware of the article you've just read, don't be surprised. With the dozens of medical journals that are published weekly or monthly, a physician could spend his entire day reading and still not keep up. But he'll do his best to stay current and will usually be aware of any truly important and proven developments in his field. The way he does that is to read a few, select journals that pertain to his particular specialty. Among them will *not* be *The National Informer.*

- *Don't* expect your doctor to have read the medical articles in the non-medical publications you've read.
- *Do* ask him his opinion about the new information you've read, but,
- *Don't* be surprised if he hasn't heard of it or doesn't feel it's reliable.

- *Don't* rely on the medical information contained in publications that also feature alien kidnappers, time travel, and four-headed cows.

The Refrigerated Stethoscope

Darryl Kwiatkowski normally didn't pay much attention to a cold. He'd take a little non-drowsy formula decongestant and some echinacea and keep right on crunching numbers in his accounting business. But this time he was miserable and had spiked a fever to 102, so he broke away from the office, even though it was late March–his busiest time of year, with the looming tax deadline–to see his physician, Dr. Margaret Claussen.

After having found Darryl's ears and throat to be clear, Dr. Claussen was trying to listen to his chest. But each time she applied her stethoscope to his skin, he wriggled away.

"Ooh," he said, "that's cold. What do you do, keep that thing in the refrigerator?"

Not hearing anything unusual in Darryl's chest so far, she gave up on listening and said, "I think it's a bad cold virus. I'll put you on something for the cough. Drink plenty of fluids–with that fever you'll need it–and get as much rest as you can. Come back if it's not getting better over the next few days."

And come back he did–the very next day, with a fever of 104 and a worsened cough. This time he was too sick to resist when she applied her stethoscope, and now she heard what she couldn't hear before: a right lower lobe pneumonia.

The cold stethoscope is a notorious instrument, but the stethoscope is designed for diagnosis, not torture. Being an inanimate object, it will take on room temperature, which, in the office environment, is going to be considerably cooler than the average temperature of 98.6 for a living human being. Since it's at least partially made of metal, it will conduct heat rapidly away from the skin, and will not stay warm long after being heated, although with repeated applications to the chest, it will warm up a bit. Certainly it can be an unpleasant sensation, but it's not painful or harmful, and it's often the anticipation of the coldness that makes the sensation worse–just like when you dip your toe into a swimming pool and then are afraid to jump into the cold water.

A closely related patient complaint is that of thin, drafty exam gowns that leave too much of the body exposed. But the whole point of an exam gown is to expose you (at least the relevant part of your anatomy), so they're rather skimpy, and they're thin because thinner is cheaper; many offices now use strictly disposable paper gowns. Offices should be kept at a reasonably comfortable temperature, but chances are it will feel a little cool to you when you're sitting resting and have just an exam gown on. The physician has on her usual clothing plus a white coat on top of that, and will be running from room to room, so she'll get overheated at a temperature that would be comfortable for you. And just like at home, there's money to be saved by turning down the thermostat.

- *Do* expect the stethoscope to feel cool to your skin, but,
- *Do* anticipate that it will be less cool as the exam continues, and,
- *Do* ask the physician to warm it up if you just can't stand it.
- *Do* put your clothing on loosely over top of the exam gown if you're cold, so it can keep you warm but still be easily removed when the physician arrives to examine you.

"Have You Ever Had This Problem, Doctor?"

Terri-Lynn Makio was in shock after receiving the news of her test results from her gynecologist, Dr. Betsy Baughman. Having had a monogamous–or so she thought—relationship with her boyfriend for nearly two years now, Terri-Lynn imagined she would be exempt from sexually transmitted diseases, and had even stopped insisting on using condoms, since she was taking birth control pills.

"The *good* news is that gonorrhea is entirely curable with antibiotics," said Dr. Baughman. "And you don't even need to get a shot nowadays; you can just take a pill."

The doctor's optimistic attitude did nothing to cheer up her patient. Terri-Lynn began sobbing and wailing.

"To think I was going to marry this guy! Now I wish he was dead–or I was dead."

Dr. Baughman touched her patient lightly on the shoulder. "I can understand your feelings…" she began.

"Oh, yeah? How would you know what I'm feeling? Have *you* ever had this problem, doctor?"

The young woman looked so miserable that her physician was moved to make a confession in sympathy. "When I was in college and engaged, I got genital herpes from my fiancé. It was difficult, but I forgave him. We got married, and eight years later we're still very happy. That's why I think I know what you're going through."

Terri-Lynn's flood of tears subsided. She took the prescription the doctor wrote for her and thanked her profusely.

Two months later, Dr. Baughman was examining another young woman, one who had recurrent, painful episodes of genital herpes. "You know," said the patient, "this used to really bum me out until I heard from my friend that you had herpes, too."

Physicians ask you all about the most intimate details of your life: your sexual habits, your drug use, your relationships. It might seem only fair that the physician should reveal herself to you as well. But the physician is asking such questions for a specific reason, in order to help diagnose and treat you, not for prurient interests. Any information she gleans is confidential (within statutory limits). Having no professional responsibility to your physician, you are not legally obligated to follow the same rules, "just" *morally*, which ought to be the higher law.

- *Don't* ask your doctor questions about her personal medical history.
- *Do* treat any information your physician may give you about her own life with the same confidentiality you would expect from her.
- *Do* realize that your doctor's decisions about her own medical care for a similar condition may not be the best for your particular problem; what worked for her may not work for you.

"Oh, My Aching Back"

Roger LeMans had been getting up with an ache in his lower back every day for the last three years, and he was getting tired of it. It wasn't bad enough to keep him from going to his job at the advertising agency, and it got better as the day wore on, but he worried that it wasn't going away. At age 35, he was surely too young to have to put up with this, he thought.

So he took a sick day and showed up in the office of Dr. Bonnie Priestley, his wife's internist. He could have sworn he saw her eyeballs roll back in her head when she opened up his chart and read the nurse's note. "So tell me about this chronic back pain you've been having," she said.

"It's been going on so long, I'm not sure where to begin. I don't know what triggered it. One day I just woke up and it was hurting. I don't remember injuring it. But there's a family history of back trouble; my dad and granddad both had bad backs, too."

"What have you tried doing about this so far?"

"I've tried a heating pad, and I've taken bottle after bottle of just about every over-the-counter pain pill. They didn't help. And I went to a massage therapist a few times, but that didn't help either."

"Well, let me give it a shot. I'll examine you and then we'll probably need to get some blood tests and X-rays and I'll see you back next week for the results."

"Next week? I thought you'd be able to take care of everything today. I'm leaving tomorrow on a two-week-long business trip to London."

This time he was sure he saw her roll her eyes.

Until now, all the chapters in this book have dealt with relationship and behavioral issues, rather than specific medical conditions that are problematic for the physician. There are however, some conditions we dread seeing on our schedules because we know the diagnosis may be elusive and the treatment may be ineffective, so the likelihood of frustration for both the patient and the physician is high. Examples include not only chronic back pain but dizziness, fatigue, and persistent headaches. This does not mean that you shouldn't go to the doctor for these problems–far from it–but when your doctor looks over your chart and sees the reason for your visit, don't be surprised if you hear a faint groan.

- *Don't* expect an instant cure for chronic backache on the first visit.

- *Do* expect that the physician may need several visits to diagnose your problem.
- *Do* expect that you may need to be referred to a sub-specialist (such as a rheumatologist, physiatrist, or orthopedist) for further evaluation.
- *Do* realize that bloodwork, X-rays, or other tests may need to be repeated if a long time has elapsed since you were first tested.
- *Do* your back exercises *regularly* if your doctor has prescribed them.
- *Do* lose weight if you're overweight; it puts extra strain on your back.

The Patient Who Plays Doctor

Harvey Harrington limped into the exam room, leaning on a walnut cane with a brass duck's head, and muttering under his breath. "Dammit, doc," said the 72-year-old retired carpenter, "I've got a kidney stone."

As the patient gingerly took a seat, Dr. Greg Fassbein said, "Tell me about what's been going on."

"It's a kidney stone, I told you," he said as he pinched his face together in pain. "My brother had the same thing and now I've got one."

"It would help if you'd describe your symptoms to me."

"The symptoms are a *kidney stone*. Can't you just give me something to help with this pain?"

"Ah, now there's a symptom: pain. Where does it hurt?"

"In my side, of course. That's where kidney stones hurt!"

"It's just that I need to make my own diagnosis, and for that I need you to tell me about your symptoms, and then I'll need to examine you and do some tests."

"Jeepers! What a waste of time, when any fool knows what a kidney stone is like!"

Dr Fassbein was nearly losing his patience. "It's not that I don't believe you, but I need to make sure for myself. So let's try again. When did your side pain start, and which side?"

"Yesterday morning when I woke up, on the right. It feels like someone's stabbing me with a knife."

"Let me take a look," Dr. Fassbein directed. When Harvey lifted his shirt, the physician knew instantly what the problem was–and it was *not* a kidney stone. A line of little blisters was beginning to form on his right mid-back–a classic case of herpes zoster. "You have 'shingles,' Mr. Harrington."

"Are you sure?" asked the bewildered patient.

"It's staring me right in the face."

"Funny. I could have sworn it was a kidney stone. Oh, well, that's the first time I've ever been wrong about anything," he said with a wink.

Playing doctor is fun when you're a kid. You make terrifying, instant diagnoses and then proceed with emergency surgery with your little plastic instruments, and have no worry about the result–if the patient dies, you just go play in the sandbox. As adults it can be fun to fantasize about being a doctor, too, as you watch television shows packed with dramatic medical situations. You need to keep in mind, though, that playing doctor for real can have real-and possibly serious-consequences.

- *Do* take care of yourself, in terms of eating right, getting some exercise, reducing stress, and avoiding harmful behaviors like smoking.

- *Do* mention to your doctor what your concerns and suspicions are regarding your possible diagnosis.

- *Don't* assume the doctor will arrive at the same conclusion as you after talking to you and examining you.

- *Do* follow the recommended treatment even if it differs from what you had expected, but let the doctor know if it's not working, and discuss any continued suspicions that you feel something else is causing the problem.

- *Don't* play doctor; let your doctor *work* at it.

Postscript

Of course, there are two sides to every relationship, and physicians sometimes need to be reminded "how to be your patients' favorite doctor." Observing these rules will also help ensure that patients get the care they deserve.

So, for all us physicians, we must remember:

- *Do* listen to your patients, allowing time for them to fully express themselves.
- *Do* address them with the name they prefer.
- *Do* use language that is appropriate for their educational level, neither talking down to them nor using overly-complicated medical jargon.
- *Do* cleanse your hands before and after examining each of your patients.
- *Do* respect your patients' modesty, allowing them to remain clothed or in a gown until it's necessary to remove them for the exam.
- *Do* apologize if you are running late—your patients' time is valuable too.
- *Do* give advice about modifying your patients' lifestyle for health purposes, but *don't* be judgmental.
- *Do* take notes during the exam, but *do* maintain eye contact with your patients most of the time, and be seated at a comfortable distance and at the same level with them.
- *Don't* treat your patients as a disease, but as a person.
- *Do* appreciate your patients; say "thank you" to *them* sometimes.

And above all, in this as in all other walks of life, *do* unto others as you would have them *do* unto you!

About the Author

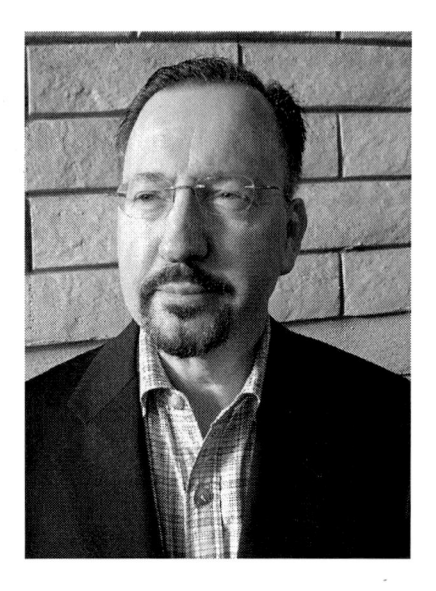

BRAD COLEGATE IS A primary care physician who graduated from the Ohio State University College of Medicine and then completed a residency in Family Medicine.

He is currently retired and enjoying other pursuits such as gardening, composing music, and reflecting on his and his patients' experiences in medical care, which resulted in the writing of this book.

About the Illustrator

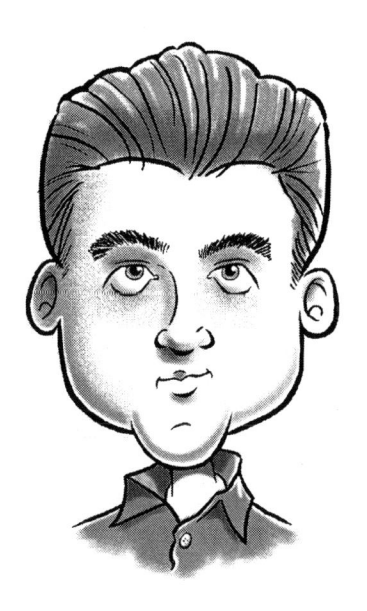

JIM CAPUTO HAS BEEN an illustrator and graphic designer for more than 25 years. After working as an art director for several ad agencies, he opened his own studio and began illustrating children's books and magazines.

In his spare time, he enjoys reading, physical fitness, going to movies, and spending time with his dog Donovan. He is a member of the Graphic Artists Guild and the Society of Children's Book Writers and Illustrators.

Published by FastPencil
http://www.fastpencil.com